THE
GOODBYE BACK AND NECK PAIN HANDBOOK

JAMES H. WHEELER, M.D. AND JAMES A. PETERSON, PH. D.

SAGAMORE PUBLISHING

CHAMPAIGN, IL

Interior Design: Michelle Summers
Cover Design: Erin Jacobs and Shawn Murdock
Editor: Susan McKinney

ISBN: 1-57167-055-6
Library of Congress Catalog Card Number: 97-68387

Sagamore Publishing
804 North Neil Street, Suite 100
Champaign, IL 61820
www.sagamorepub.com

Printed in the United States.

To our wives—Sandee and Susan—whose support, love and guidance in our lives provided us with motivation to help others by writing this book.

—and—

To James and Virginia Wheeler, whose upbringing laid the groundwork for the educational, personal and professional successes their son, James H. Wheeler M.D. has been so fortunate to enjoy.

ACKNOWLEDGMENTS

We have had numerous opportunities in our lifetimes to work in an environment and with colleagues who by their presence serve as continuing sources of motivation and inspiration. We would like to express our appreciation to these individuals for the impact that they have had on our professional lives and on our efforts to write this book. We would also like to thank Peter Bannon, President of Sagamore Publishing, Inc., for his efforts in enabling this book to be published.

CONTENTS

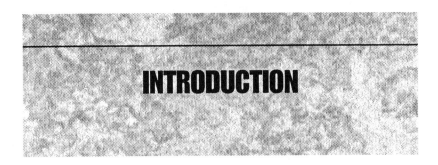

INTRODUCTION

"Your lot is mortal: not mortal is what you desire."
—Ovid

Each of us became deeply involved with the treatment and prevention of back and neck pain in a different way. One became involved as a natural outgrowth of his professional responsibilities as a trained orthopedic surgeon. In that position, he has seen hundreds of patients suffering from back and neck pain. The other became interested nearly 17 years ago when he first suffered a bout of back pain. Quite frankly, before his unwelcomed initiation into the world of back pain, he had never given the matter much thought.

With our diverse backgrounds and perspectives, some may wonder how we got together to share ideas on treating back pain and why we undertook the collaborative effort that resulted in this book. The answer to both questions is relatively simple: During the mid-to-late 1980s we shared a mutual concern for the health and welfare of the members of the West Point community—the cadets, staff and faculty, support personnel and dependents. Despite the strong community-wide emphasis on fitness and wellness, West Point had a pattern of serious back pain suffering similar to that in most communities. Even among the Corps of Cadets—probably the most physically fit college-age student body anywhere—the incidence of back pain was relatively great. Moreover, the intense physical demands of a career as an officer in the United States Army made such a condition even more intolerable. As a result, we both spent considerable effort and energy in an attempt to better understand the causes of back pain so that we might be able to identify more effective and efficient methods for dealing with it.

As you will read in this book, medicine is not an exact science. Understandably, this is not the best news for those who suffer from back or neck pain. If members of the medical community cannot agree on what is wrong with back and neck pain sufferers and how to treat them, is it any wonder that literally millions of back and neck pain sufferers face what they perceive to be a hopeless situation?

This book was developed in an attempt to at least partially rectify that dilemma. Actually, this second edition of *The Goodbye Back and Neck Pain Handbook* was written to serve three objectives. *First,* we want to provide an overview of the basic information you should know about your spine. Certainly, more technical and more comprehensive explanations of how the spine works and why it may not work properly have been penned. At some point, however, the information can become so complex and so overbearing as to divert your willingness or ability to adequately comprehend what you are reading. For those who would like a thorough description of the anatomy of the spine, the bibliography at the end of the book provides suggestions for additional reading material. *Second,* the book attempts to crack the veneer of hopelessness facing many back and neck pain sufferers. Your back and neck pain can and should be treated. This book is an essential first step in that treatment. *Third,* this book provides an overview of the various Tempur-Pedic products and a discussion of how the features of these innovative products can help back and neck pain sufferers.

Chapter 1 presents an overview of the anatomy of the spine. Chapter 2 offers a synopsis of the most common causes of back and neck pain. An explanation of how back and neck pain are diagnosed and evaluated is included in Chapter 3. Chapter 4 discusses how individuals can treat their back and neck pain. An overview of the various Tempur-Pedic products for treating and preventing back and neck pain is presented in Chapter 5. Chapter 6 offers common-sense suggestions on how best to prevent back and neck pain from occurring. Finally, Chapter 7 includes some of the most commonly asked questions regarding back and neck pain and the answers to each inquiry.

It is certainly a natural inclination, before reading further, to ask yourself the following question: "Will reading this book and following the advice included in it guarantee that my back or neck will get better?" In all honesty, no one—including the two of us—can make that guarantee. What we've presented in this book is our best opinion, based upon the most current information available and our years of firsthand experience with those who suffer from back and neck pain. While we feel strongly that the information in this book is the best advice we can offer, ultimately you must assume full responsibility for whatever course of action you decide to take. If our advice differs from that of your doctor, we suggest that you either follow the suggestions of your own physician, who obviously has the advantage of having examined you and knowing your unique situation, or consult another doctor for another opinion.

Other than accentuating your feelings of relief when you're not experiencing it, back and neck pain have absolutely no redeeming value. *The Goodbye Back and Neck Pain Handbook* was written to enable you to say, "Goodbye back and neck pain, hello life."

Simply reading this book, however, won't make your pain go away. Despite the mild disclaimer in the previous paragraph, we strongly recommend that you follow the suggestions we offer in this book. Keep in mind that if you sincerely want your back and neck pain to "go away," it is absolutely critical that you closely adhere to proper techniques for caring for your spine. Mix in a reasonable measure of common sense and a dash of plain old hard work, and you've got a great chance to succeed. We wish you luck.

James Wheeler, M.D., FAAOS, FACS
James A. Peterson, Ph.D., FACSM

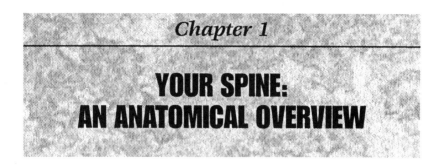

Chapter 1

YOUR SPINE: AN ANATOMICAL OVERVIEW

"If anything is sacred, the human body is sacred."
—Walt Whitman

When someone is called the "backbone" of an organization, it is obvious that that individual is vital to the health and well-being of that organization. Similarly, the human backbone (spine) is vital to the health and well-being of each person. Your spine is the basic *support* system that connects your upper body with your lower body, allowing you to sit, stand upright, work, walk, run and jump. It also serves the important function of *protection* for your spinal cord. In addition to support and protection, the spine is flexible so that *motion* can occur. Providing support, protection and the flexibility for motion, your spine easily qualifies as one of the most vital components of your good health and well-being (Figure 1-1).

When this vital component is not working and causes you pain and distress, you obviously want to know why, and you want to know what you can do to remedy the situation. However, before you can understand why your back or neck doesn't work properly, you must understand how they are supposed to function, and that requires some knowledge of the anatomy of the spine. Your spine is made of many parts, all working together. A problem with any one of the individual parts can lead to dysfunction of your entire spine.

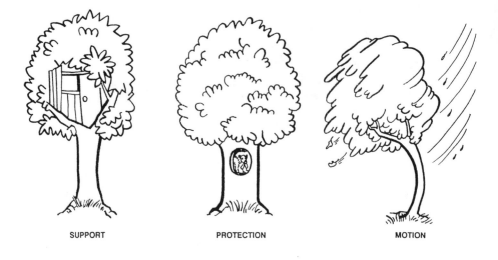

SUPPORT   PROTECTION   MOTION

Figure 1-1   Functions of the backbone

The spine has three basic components: 1) the bony framework (bones, ligaments and discs), 2) the spinal cord (and nerves) and 3) the muscles. By becoming familiar with the anatomy of the basic parts of your spine, you will be better able to understand how each component functions individually and how all the components function together.

THE BONY FRAMEWORK: BONES, DISCS AND LIGAMENTS

Bones

Your spine is made up of 24 individual bones located between your skull and your pelvis, plus the sacrum and the coccyx (Figure 1-2). These bones are called vertebrae and are connected by discs and ligaments. The vertebrae are named according to their location in the spine. The upper seven vertebrae are known as the cervical vertebrae of the neck (C1-C7), and the lower five vertebrae are called the lumbar vertebrae of the lower back (L1-L5). In between are the 12 thoracic vertebrae, to which the ribs are attached (T1-T12).

The lowest lumbar vertebrae (L5) sits on top of your sacrum. The sacrum is a broad, triangular, bony structure composed of five vertebrae that fused together into a single bone during the first few months of your life. The sacrum is designed to provide rigid support for your pelvis. Your coccyx is a collection of three or four small vertebrae fused into a single vertebra. It is frequently referred to as the "tailbone," since it is probably the remnant of what once was mankind's tail. About two inches long, your coccyx attaches to the lower point of your sacrum. It provides an anchorage for several of the small muscles in your rectal area that are essential to the control of bowel movement.

When viewed from behind, your spine should be straight (Figure 1-2). When viewed from the side, the vertebrae are aligned so that your spine has a gentle lazy S curve to it. This curve is formed by a forward bend of your spine in the cervical and lumbar areas and a backward bend in the thoracic area. These curves balance each other so that your head is centered over your pelvis.

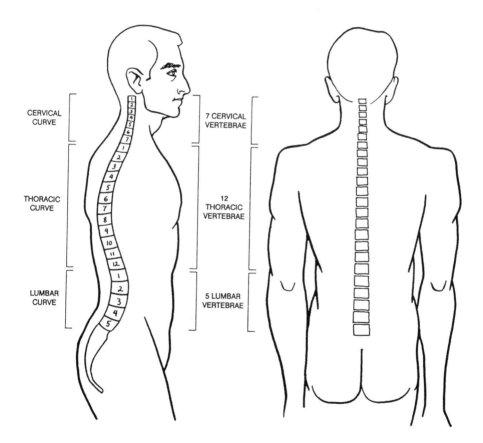

Figure 1-2   The spine: side and back views

The vertebrae form a protective ring around the spinal cord. The center of this ring is called the spinal canal because it is the canal through which your spinal cord passes. The anatomy of this protective ring can be best appreciated by looking at an individual vertebra from above (Figure 1-3). The ring of bone is formed by the vertebral body in front, the pedicles on the side and the lamina in back. Each vertebra also has a spinous process and two transverse processes to which ligaments, muscles and ribs attach. Looking at a vertebra from the side, you can see that each vertebra is connected to the vertebra above and below it by its facet joints and by a disc. The opening on the side of each vertebra is for the spinal nerves to exit the protective bony framework of the spine.

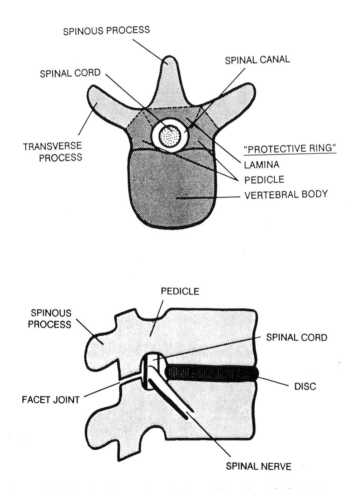

Figure 1-3   Vertebra: from above (top) and from the side (bottom).

Discs

Discs are structures between adjoining vertebrae. "Disc" is an appropriate descriptive term because each disc has a flat, circular shape (Figure 1-4). Discs are made of cartilage material similar in consistency to rubber, and they function as the shock absorbers of the spine.

Each disc has a semisolid center (nucleus) that is supported by a ring of tissue (annulus) that surrounds this center. The center of the disc is mainly responsible for the shock absorbing properties of the disc, and the ring of tissue is the support that prevents the disc from collapsing.

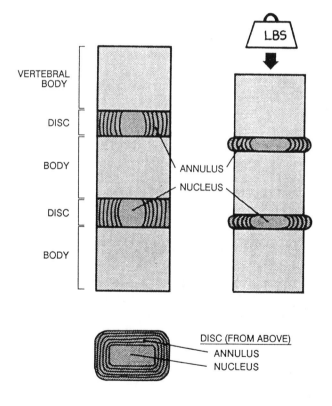

Figure 1-4   Two side views of discs, illustrating their shock-absorbing properties, and a disc viewed from above

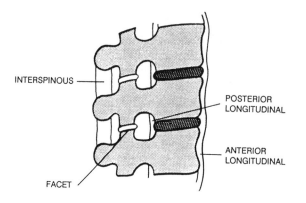

Figure 1-5   Ligaments of the spine

Ligaments

Ligaments are strong bands of fibrous connective tissue that function to hold bones together. Each joint in your body is formed by two bones held together by ligaments. Whereas ligaments are strong enough to hold joints together, they are also flexible and elastic enough to allow controlled motion in a joint. If a ligament is torn, however, excessive motion can occur, and a joint can be dislocated.

In the spine, the ligaments function to hold the vertebrae together, and there are several ligaments in your spine that connect each vertebra to the one above and below it (Figure 1-5). The only direct bone-to-bone connection between adjoining vertebrae is the facet joints, which are held together by ligaments. Although there is some motion between the vertebral bodies where they come into contact with the discs, it is at the facet joints where the majority of spinal motion occurs. The connection of the vertebral bodies to each other through the disc is supported by the anterior and posterior longitudinal ligaments. These ligaments extend from the top of your spine down to your sacrum, with one at the front and the other at the back of the vertebral body. The posterior ligament separates the bodies of the vertebrae from your spinal canal. Additional stability is provided by the interspinous ligaments, which extend from the spinous process of one vertebrae to the spinous process of the next, down the entire length of your spine, and by the ligamentum flavum, which connects lamina to lamina.

THE SPINAL CORD

Your spinal cord is a direct extension of your brain and is responsible for carrying messages from your brain to your body and from your body back to your brain (Figure 1-6). These messages are transmitted through nerves in a fashion similar to the conduction of electricity through telephone wires. A nerve has two basic functions: motor and sensory. The motor nerves are responsible for activating muscle groups or organs to perform certain actions. The sensory nerves provide input to your brain from your body. The combination of sensory input and motor output allows your body (using its brain, spinal cord and nerves) to respond appropriately to external stimuli.

To illustrate sensory and motor interactions, consider the following example. If you touch a hot stove with your hand, a sensory nerve takes that information to your spinal cord, which transmits it to your brain. Your brain then interprets that information and sends a message down through your spinal cord to a motor nerve, which activates the muscle group that pulls your hand away from the stove. You can appreciate how fast this sensory input and motor output process occurs when you consider how quickly you pull your hand away from the stove.

The human nervous system (brain, spinal cord and nerves) is magnificent in the way it works, but it is also very fragile and needs very good protection. The skull is made of hard bone to protect your brain, and the backbone protects your spinal cord.

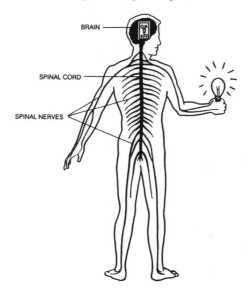

Figure 1-6 The brain, spinal cord and nerves

THE SPINAL MUSCLES

The 140 muscles that run along the back of your spine from the base of your skull to your pelvis and attach to your spine are called the spinal muscles. These muscles perform a substantial amount of work. Other muscles aid the spinal muscles in supporting your spine. The abdominal muscles are very important in supporting your spine, much more so than most people realize. They are so important that they could be considered the "anterior spinal muscles." The muscles of your pelvis, hips and upper legs, including the buttock, hamstring and quadriceps muscles also directly or indirectly support your spine.

The framework of your spine is provided by the vertebral bones held together by ligaments and discs, but it is your muscles that support that framework and provide the means for motion (Figure 1-7). If, for example, you become paralyzed, even though your bones and ligaments are functional, you will be unable to stand erect because you do not have functioning muscles. Similarly, when you faint, you will fall to the ground because all your muscles have stopped working momentarily. Muscles and the voluntary control that you have over them give you the ability to stand erect and move about.

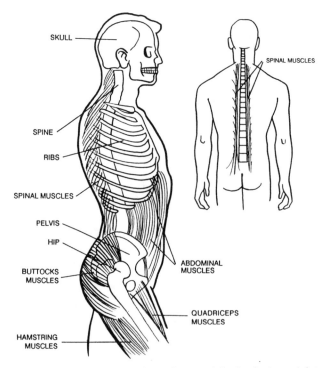

Figure 1-7   The spinal muscles: side view (left), back view (right)

FUNCTION

As stated before, your spine is a well-constructed system that connects and supports your upper and your lower body, provides protection for your spinal cord, but yet allows flexibility and motion. For these functions of support, protection and motion to be effectively and painlessly accomplished, all the components of your spine must be in good working order.

The bones in your back and neck are the foundation or building blocks of your spine, held together by ligaments and discs, with motion occurring from the action of your muscles. A healthy spine is sturdy and strong for support and protection, but it is also flexible so that motion can occur.

THE NEXT STEP

The preceding section on the anatomy of your spine was designed to provide you with an abbreviated overview of how your back and neck work. Chapter 2 examines the causes of back and neck pain. We recommend that when necessary, you refer back to this chapter for an explanation of basic spine anatomy. The effort will be worthwhile. Comprehending what is wrong with your back or neck and what to do about it will be easier if you understand how your spine normally functions.

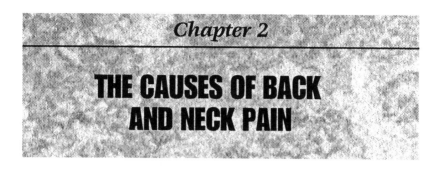

Chapter 2

THE CAUSES OF BACK AND NECK PAIN

"Your cause is hidden but the result is well known."

—Ovid

Humans are more prone to back and neck pain than four-legged animals, because they stand in an upright position and transmit the gravitational forces on their spines to two legs rather than four legs. This increase of the natural forces of gravity is concentrated in the lower neck and the lower back area. Understandably, it is the lower cervical spine that is the source of most neck pain and the lower lumbar spine that is the source of most back pain.

To understand what causes back and neck pain, you must have an insight into the spine's anatomy. Briefly, your vertebral bones are the framework of the spine that protects your spinal cord and the nerves coming from it. Your vertebrae are held together by ligaments and discs, and the motion of the vertebrae is controlled by muscles. Problems with any one of these structures (vertebrae, ligaments, discs, muscles, spinal cord or nerves) can cause back or neck pain. This chapter examines the common and the not-so-common causes of back and neck pain and attempts to explain why some people have back or neck pain with no apparent cause.

CATEGORIZING BACK AND NECK PAIN

Back and neck pain have not traditionally been described and categorized in a number of ways. We recommend categorizing back and neck pain on the basis of two broad parameters. The system we advocate is based on an attempt to simplify the description and categorization process for back and neck pain in terms that most individuals can understand.

First, we describe pain by the length of time it has been present. Back or neck pain that started recently (days, to a few weeks ago) is termed acute, and pain of a repetitive, long-standing nature is called chronic.

Second, we further describe pain by the basic mechanism causing the pain without referring to any specific anatomical structure. There are two basic mechanisms of back pain: traumatic and degenerative. Traumatic infers that some injury or injuries are the basic cause of the pain, whereas degenerative indicates that arthritis or the normal aging process is the primary cause of the pain. Although there are many other, less common causes of back and neck pain (some of which will be discussed later in this chapter), the two most common mechanisms are traumatic and degenerative.

Explaining pain when there is no mechanism or cause is not as easy. We use the term idiopathic to define back or neck pain that apparently normal people have when there is no obvious reason for the pain and when the other causes of pain have been excluded.

Back and neck pain, then, can be grouped into four basic categories: 1) traumatic, 2) degenerative, 3) idiopathic and 4) other. Table 2-1 is a listing of the basic categories of back and neck pain and includes examples of the basic causes of pain associated with each category. Traumatic, degenerative and idiopathic pain are discussed in some detail in subsequent sections, followed by an abbreviated overview of several of the causes designated as other pain.

---

1. TRAUMATIC PAIN
- Fractured bones
- Sprained ligaments
- Strained muscles
- Disc injuries

2. DEGENERATIVE PAIN
- Degenerative arthritis
- Degenerative discs
- Spinal stenosis

3. IDIOPATHIC PAIN
- "Everyday" back pain in healthy people
- Poor posture—excess weight
- Pregnancy
- Overuse injuries
- Poor flexibility—hamstring tightness

4. OTHER CAUSES OF PAIN
- Developmental (scoliosis, kyphosis, lordosis, spondylolisthesis)
- Inflammatory (rheumatoid arthritis, ankylosing spondylitis)
- Infection
- Neoplastic (tumors)
- Metabolic (osteoporosis)

Table 2-1   Causes of back and neck pain

TRAUMATIC BACK AND NECK PAIN

Everyone can relate to fractured wrist bones, sprained ankle ligaments and a strained leg muscle. These types of injuries can also occur in the bones, ligaments and muscles of your back, either singly or in combination with one another. Unfortunately, we are not as familiar with our back as we are with our arms and legs (we need a mirror just to see our back or the back of our neck). For this reason, we sometimes have difficulty understanding that a sprained or injured back or neck can be caused by the same things that cause a sprained or injured leg muscle. In addition, traumatic back or neck pain can be caused by discs that rupture or herniate.

Any injury can be acute, which means that the injury recently occurred. On the other hand, an injury can be chronic in nature, meaning that over the months or years, several or many injuries have occurred. A chronic injury may be a significant injury but, more commonly, it is an accumulation of milder injuries.

Fractured Bones

Just as you can fall and fracture bones in your wrist, you can also fracture the bones of your spine (vertebrae). Thankfully, however, fractures of the vertebrae are not nearly as common as fractures of other bones in your body. In fact, fractures of the spinal bones are unusual in healthy people, and they occur most often as a result of a significant injury, such as a bad fall or a car accident.

Your spine is a very well-constructed support system that can absorb a great deal of shock or impact without fracturing the bones because the discs be-tween the vertebrae pro-tect the bones of the spine. You can imagine how fragile we would be without these built-in shock absorbers. Injuries to the discs are far more common than fractures of the spine. This is important to know, because a fracture of your spine that causes a displacement or shattering of the bones could lead to an injury to your spinal cord and possible paralysis.

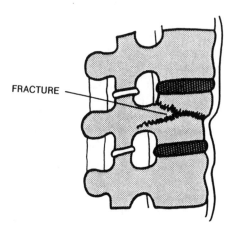

FRACTURE

Figure 2-1   A fractured bone

Sprained Ligaments and Strained Muscles

The most common injuries of the spine are not injuries to the bones or discs but rather injuries to the ligaments (sprains) and muscles (strains). The mechanisms of sprained ligaments and strained muscles in the spine are similar to the mechanisms of injuries that occur elsewhere in the body. For example, athletes can strain a leg muscle running, or they can strain a back muscle while lifting too much. Basketball players can twist and sprain their ankles, or they can twist and sprain their backs. Because the ligaments and muscles of your spine are so close to each other, however, it may not be as easy to differentiate between injuries to the ligaments and injuries to the muscles of your back or neck as it is elsewhere in your body.

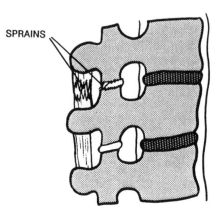

SPRAINS

Figure 2-2   Sprained ligaments

A sprained ligament occurs when it is stretched beyond its normal fixed length, such as can happen with sudden or violent bending or twisting. When you use your back to lift or move, motion occurs between each vertebra. The ligaments function as check-reins or tie-downs to prevent excessive motion. When the maximum allowable motion has occurred, the ligament becomes taut. The ligaments have some elasticity and the ability to stretch a small amount, but not a great deal. A sprained ligament can vary from very mild to severe. A sprain is classified as mild when there is no significant damage to the ligament. In a mild sprain, pain occurs when that ligament is stretched, although the pain may not be present until the day after the injury. A severe sprain means that the ligament has been damaged or torn. In this instance the pain will be much worse and recovery longer. When an injury occurs to a ligament in your spine, any motion of that injured area will stress the injured ligament and be very painful. As a result, your sprained back or neck becomes stiff and painful to move.

If a ligament has been torn, it will heal, but it may not be as taut as it was originally. Part of the healing process includes the formation of scar tissue, which is not as strong as normal ligamentous tissue and is less flexible. A healed torn ligament usually is not as tight, not as strong and not as flexible as an uninjured ligament and that ligament is more likely to be reinjured and probably will be. Also, the scar tissue formed as part of the healing process can be a source of chronic pain.

A strained muscle ("pulled muscle," "charley horse") most often occurs when a muscle is stressed beyond its capability to contract, such as when a back muscle is strained when you lift something too heavy or lift something in an improper manner. A muscle strain can also occur when a relaxed or partially relaxed muscle is suddenly or unexpectedly overstretched. Whereas ligaments have a relatively fixed length, the length of a muscle changes markedly depending on the degree of contraction. The ability to voluntarily contract or relax skeletal muscles gives you the ability to control the motion in your joints.

Muscle strains vary from mild to severe depending on the amount of damage to the muscle unit. In a mild strain, there is no appreciable damage to the muscle, and, although the muscle is able to function, you experience pain when you use it. The pain may not occur until the day following the injury after the muscle has tightened or stiffened up. In a severe strain, there is a tear of the muscles that is accompanied by significant pain and dysfunction.

A muscle spasm may occur after a muscle has been injured. A muscle tightens up, or goes into spasm, as a way of protecting itself from further overstretching and further injury. Muscle spasm can also occur after another structure near the muscle (a ligament, bone or disc) has been injured. This muscle spasm occurs because the muscles become secondarily irritated by the injury or because the muscles are trying to protect the injured area. When a muscle goes into spasm, motion around that injured area is decreased, protecting that area from further injury and from motion that would be painful.

As a muscle strain heals, the pain and spasm associated with it will subside. If there has been a tear in the muscle, the healing process includes formation of some scar tissue in the injured area. The scar tissue formed is not as elastic as normal muscle tissue, and the muscle may lose some of its ability to relax and contract. This loss of elasticity makes that muscle more prone to future injury. The scar tissue formed may also be a source of chronic pain in the healing or healed muscle, just as scar tissue can be a source of pain in a healing or healed ligament injury.

Proper conditioning and stretching out before and after physical activity make muscles less prone to injury. Most competitive athletes are aware not only of the benefits, but also of the necessities of proper training and stretching techniques in preventing muscle strains.

Once a muscle has been injured, conditioning and stretching are even more important in preventing future injuries.

Disc Injuries

Many terms are used in discussing disc injuries, including "slipped," "bulging," "ruptured" and "herniated." You should not be confused by these different terms, as each term is a fairly accurate description of what has actually happened to the disc.

A slipped or bulging disc is a disc that has slipped out or is bulging from between the vertebrae (Figure 2-3). A ruptured disc is a disc in which the supporting ring of tissue around the center of the disc has been disrupted. If the injury is carried one step further, the disc material in the center of the disc can herniate through the rupture in the supporting ring of tissue (Figure 2-4).

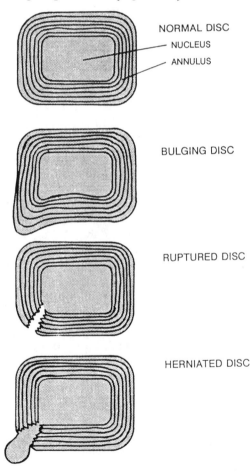

Figure 2-3   Disc injuries

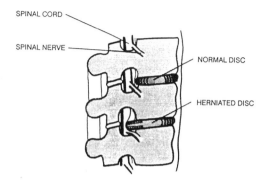

Figure 2-4   A herniated disc

An injury to the disc itself (and the ligaments supporting it) can be a source of pain. If the disc ruptures and disc material herniates, pain can come not only from the area of the injured disc but also from the disc material pressing on the spinal cord on the surrounding nerves. When a nerve gets irritated, the pain is usually sharp and intense and can be an electric-type shooting pain. If the nerve becomes irritated or pinched enough, numbness or weakness can result.

The nerve most commonly affected in lower back disc injuries is the sciatic nerve. When a herniated disc puts pressure on the sciatic nerve, the nerve becomes irritated and sciatica results. Sciatica is pain that starts in your lower back and travels along the course of the sciatic nerve through your buttocks and the back of your leg to your foot. An injury to a disc in the neck (usually the lower part of the neck) will cause pain that starts in your neck and goes to your shoulder, arm and even your hand.

DEGENERATIVE BACK AND NECK PAIN

Unfortunately, the spine, especially the lower cervical spine and the lower lumbar spine, goes through a normal aging or degeneration process that is probably accelerated in animals walking on two, rather than four, legs. Just as "old age" arthritis sets up in our knees or hips, it can also affect the bones of the spine. In fact, if several elderly individuals were to have an X-ray made of the lumbar region of the spine, most, if not all, would have at least some degenerative arthritic changes present on that X-ray. This doesn't mean, however, that all of these individuals have back pain. What it does mean is that the degenerative process involving the bones and discs is part of the normal aging process.

Degenerative Arthritis

Degenerative arthritis of the vertebral bones is similar to the "wear and tear" arthritis that occurs in other joints of your body. With this wear and tear comes inflammation, to which your body may respond by producing bone spurs. This inflammation and bone spur formation can be a source of pain in themselves or can cause pain by irritating other structures of your spine, such as the ligaments, muscles, spinal cord or surrounding nerves.

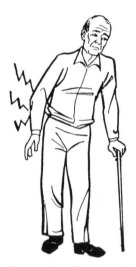

Degenerative arthritis in the spine occurs in the joints of the spine, primarily in the facet joints and between the vertebral bodies. The pain of degenerative arthritis in your spine is similar to arthritic pain in other joints of your body. This pain is occasionally sharp, but more often it is dull and aching. Arthritic pain

Figure 2-5   Characteristic stance of a person with degenerative arthritis

is aggravated by cold weather or weather changes. Since arthritic pain is also aggravated by inactivity, it is common to experience pain and stiffness in the mornings.

Degenerative Discs

Degenerative discs and degenerative arthritis of the spine usually accompany each other. The degenerative aging process that affects the vertebrae also affects their shock absorbers, the discs. The discs are made of a cartilage substance similar in consistency to hard rubber. With increasing age, the water content of these discs decreases and, as a result, the discs flatten and lose their shock absorbing capacity (Figure 2-6). A disc degenerates slowly over a period of time. A degenerative disc usually is referred to as a flattened or bulging disc, not as a ruptured or herniated disc that is traumatic in origin.

The pain of a degenerative disc is similar to the dull, aching pain of degenerative arthritis. A degenerative disc can put pressure on your spinal cord and nerves. Because the formation of a degenerative disc is such a gradual process, however, you may not remember when you initially experienced the pain. The leg pain of a degenerative disc is not as sharp or well-defined as the pain of sciatica (the sharp pain felt down your leg) from a herniated disc. Those with a herniated disc can usually remember the day their sciatic pain started, but those with a degenerative disc will speak in months or years when asked when their back or leg pain started.

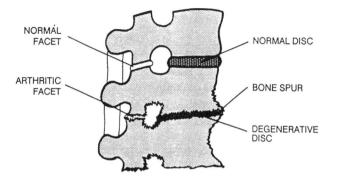

Figure 2-6   Causes of degenerative spine pain: degenerative arthritis and degenerative discs

Spinal Stenosis

Spinal stenosis is the term that is used to describe the narrowing of the spinal canal (carrying the spinal cord and nerves). Any condition that narrows the spinal canal (a herniated disc, for example) is, in effect, spinal stenosis (Figure 2-7). The term spinal stenosis, however, usually refers to the narrowing of the spinal canal that is associated with degenerative arthritis and degenerative discs.

Spinal stenosis is a degenerative process associated with aging. Not surprisingly, most patients with spinal stenosis are over age 50. The arthritis that is present in the facet joints and between the vertebral bodies causes bone spur formation. This arthritis, along with degenerative bulging discs, combines to narrow the cross sectional area of the spinal canal and put pressure on the spinal cord and nerves.

A combination of back and leg pain (or neck and arm pain) is the result of spinal stenosis. The back pain is similar to the chronic, aching pain of degenerative arthritis. The leg pain is similar to the leg pain associated with degenerative discs and is

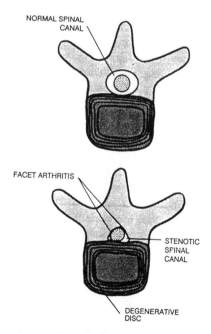

Figure 2-7   Spinal stenosis

caused by pressure on the spinal cord and nerves. The leg pain of spinal stenosis may be quite vague. It is sometimes blamed on poor circulation because it comes on after physical activity. If you experience spinal stenosis, you soon learn how far you can walk before your legs start hurting and how long they take to stop hurting when you rest.

Spinal stenosis is suspected when someone over the age of 50 has a somewhat vague history of back and leg (or neck and arm) pain, doesn't have any dramatic physical findings on examination, but does have arthritis on regular X-rays. The diagnosis is confirmed by a computerized tomography (CT or CAT) scan, a myelogram, or magnetic resonance imaging (MRI). See chapter 3 for an explanation of these tests.

IDIOPATHIC BACK AND NECK PAIN ("EVERYDAY" PAIN IN HEALTHY PEOPLE)

It is easy to understand why someone has back or neck pain after they have had an injury to their spine. It is also relatively easy to explain to elderly individuals that their back or neck pain is caused by arthritis in their spine. It is not so easy, however, to explain why healthy, young individuals have back pain when they are physically fit and have never had a back injury.

Unfortunately, it is "normal" for healthy, young people to have back or neck pain at some point, and, in fact, almost everyone has experienced or will experience back or neck pain during their lifetime. About one-half of the working force is unable to go to work because of back or neck pain at some time in their lives.

The previous sections discussed traumatic and degenerative back and neck pain. The third, and perhaps most common, grouping of back and neck pain is idiopathic. This category concerns pain in otherwise fit and healthy people.

Idiopathic is a word that means "no known cause." The term "idiopathic back pain" is used to categorize that group of people who have back pain, but don't have a good reason for it and don't fall into one of the other three categories of back pain (traumatic, degenerative or other). There are several factors in idiopathic back or neck pain that may predispose an otherwise healthy person to pain. These include the effects of poor posture and excess weight, pregnancy, overuse injuries and poor flexibility and tight hamstring muscles.

Sleeping is another significant factor in "everyday" back and neck pain in normal healthy people. How good or bad your back and neck feel after sleeping and other factors affecting back and neck pain will be discussed on the next several pages.

Poor Posture and Excess Weight

Poor posture or excess weight alone may not cause back or neck pain overnight, nor will they necessarily ever cause pain. Long-standing poor posture and excess weight, however, increase the forces on your spine and can accelerate the degenerative changes that are inevitable with age. As mentioned previously, humans walking on two legs in an upright position already have more forces placed on their spine than do four-legged animals.

The human spine when viewed from the side curves in a gentle, lazy S shape. Poor posture and excess weight increase the curves that are normally present, causing kyphosis (an increase in the thoracic curve) and lordosis (an increase in the lumbar curve). Changing the spinal curves increases the forces and stresses on your vertebrae, discs, ligaments and muscles (Figure 2-8).

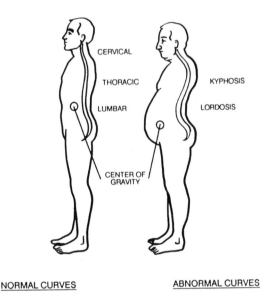

Figure 2-8   The effects of poor posture and excess weight

Prolonged bad posture and excess weight also place all of the components of your spine at risk for injury and pain. Because your vertebrae and discs have increased forces put on them, they are more susceptible to degenerative changes. Your ligaments also incur increased stresses. As a result, they are more prone to chronic injury. Your muscles are put at a mechanical disadvantage, forcing them to work harder to accomplish the same amount of work or causing them to become lazy in the position of poor posture. Either way, they are more prone to chronic injury.

Those who don't think that excess weight or a big, protruding belly can aggravate or cause back pain should fill their pockets with lead, strap a bowling ball to their belly and wear a backpack every day for several years. Not only will their back likely hurt, but so will their hips, knees and ankles.

Pregnancy

Pregnancy is an example of an increase in abdominal weight that causes a change in posture, increases forces on the spine and predisposes the pregnant female to back pain. Placing the pregnant female in the same category as the overweight poor-postured individual is not quite fair but, however, as far as the spine is concerned, the same basic process is occurring during the pregnancy.

The excess lower abdominal weight, especially later in the pregnancy, has a similar effect on the spine as excess weight and poor posture in nonpregnant people. The additional weight causes an increase in the curve normally present in the lumbar spine (lordosis). The change in this curve and the additional body weight places increased forces and stresses on the vertebrae, discs, ligaments and muscles of the spine. As a result, the components of the spine are more susceptible to fatigue, injury and pain.

Back pain does not necessarily accompany pregnancy, but pregnancy does place the back at an increased risk for pain. If you experienced back pain before and become pregnant, the chances are even greater that you will have more back pain during your pregnancy.

Overuse Injuries

Overuse injuries in athletes, especially runners, are a well-known problem. Because we are not as familiar with the anatomy or function of our back as we are of our extremities, it is not as well-understood or accepted why we can get overuse problems with our back.

All parts of our body, including our spine, have a certain limit of activity that they can endure before problems arise. Different people have different limits, but everyone eventually reaches the point of overuse. Conditioned marathon runners may not reach this limit until they are running 25 miles every day, whereas individuals just starting a running program may encounter problems after running their first mile. Most of you can remember your healthy years as a child when you could play outside all day long every day. Now, as a weekend athlete, you often go to work on Mondays painfully sore from the activities of your weekend.

If weekend athletes have back or neck pain on Mondays, it is usually because they have overused the muscles and other spinal components on the weekend that they had underused the rest of the week. Overuse and underuse are terms relative to whatever "normal" use is. As a "normally active" person, you are susceptible to overuse injuries from athletics. You are also susceptible to overuse injuries in your back and neck from the activities of daily life, including sitting, standing, walking, bending and lifting. A common overuse back or neck pain is the pain that the secretary-typist gets from sitting at her desk all day long. Sitting with an erect, rigid spine stresses the muscles and other components of the spine, eventually causing fatigue, stiffness and pain.

Listing possible overuse problems of the spine is an endless task. Everyone—the weekend athlete, the everyday athlete, the white collar or blue collar worker—is a potential victim of back or neck pain from overuse or underuse. A strong and healthy spine needs to be used to remain strong and healthy. You should remember, however, that there is a fine line between using your back, overusing it and underusing it.

Poor Flexibility, Hamstring Tightness, and Back Pain

For any muscle or joint to be healthy and functioning, it needs to be strong and flexible. This applies to your back, the muscles of your back and the muscles that directly or indirectly support your back—especially your hamstring muscles. A vicious cycle can begin and perpetuate itself when a normal muscle or joint is just a little stiff and sore from being used or has a minor injury. In order to protect this muscle or joint, you don't use it through its normal range of motion. When you eventually do try to use it, it is still sore because it is still stiff. As time goes on, it becomes more stiff (loses flexibility), becomes more difficult to function normally and becomes more prone to injury, which causes more loss of flexibility, more loss of function and so on. As you can see, a vicious cycle is set in motion.

Flexibility plays an important part in recovering from back pain and in preventing back pain from recurring. Following an episode of back pain, no matter what the cause, you must regain the flexibility in your back and hamstring muscles so that your back can function normally. If you do not restore your level of flexibility, your back will not function normally and will be more prone to future problems, including the recurrence of back pain.

There are some of us who are normally very flexible ("double jointed"), just as there are some of us who are not very flexible. The young gymnast can bend over and touch her palms to the floor without difficulty, but the husky young weightlifter may be able to bend over and only touch his fingertips to his knees. Does an inherent lack of flexibility make someone more prone to back pain? And, if someone has back pain and a lack of flexibility, which condition came first? Did the lack of flexibility cause the back pain, or did the pain cause the lack of flexibility? Regardless of which came first, lack of flexibility or back pain, it is obvious that they are closely related, because often when one disappears, so will the other.

A common problem in people with low back pain is tightness of the hamstring muscles, the powerful muscles in the back of the thigh. A measure commonly used to evaluate back pain is the straight leg test (discussed further in Chapter 3). In this test you lie flat on your back with your legs straight. The doctor then lifts one of your legs off the table and raises it as far as possible. Normally, your leg should be able to be raised to an angle of 90 degrees from the horizontal. Problems that cause a limit in the straight leg test include back pain, disc problems and tight hamstrings. This test demonstrates the interrelationship between back pain and tight hamstrings.

Lack of flexibility in your hamstring muscles can by itself be a significant contributing factor to back pain, or it can be secondary to the pain in your back. Either way, maintaining or gaining flexibility in your hamstring muscles is an important part of the prevention or treatment of back pain. Stretching exercises for the hamstring muscles and other muscle groups are shown in Chapter 6.

SLEEPING AND BACK/NECK PAIN

Sleeping, especially a good night's sleep, is a very important part of your life, not only from an overall health and well-being standpoint but also for the care and prevention of back and neck pain. Everyone would like to get a good night's sleep, wake up rested, refreshed, comfortable and ready to go. Too often, we don't get a good night's sleep and wake up restless, tired, stiff and dreading the day ahead. Considering that we spend about eight hours a day or one-third of our total lives sleeping or trying to sleep, it should be apparent to us the importance of a good night's sleep, especially if you have back or neck pain.

There are several reasons why sleeping can cause, aggravate or relieve back and neck pain. These include the amount of time we spend relatively inactive on a sleeping surface (mattress and pillow) that may or may not conform to the shape of our spine and may cause or relieve pressure on parts of our body. Finding a mattress and pillow that conforms to the shape of our spine and relieves pressure on the spine and other body parts, should lead to a better night's sleep and relief or prevention of back and neck pain.

If your back or neck or any other part of your body is sore at the end of a day, simply because it or you is tired or worn out, a good night's rest will make it and you feel better. On the other hand, even normal muscles and joints will stiffen with inactivity, which includes the relative inactivity of sleeping eight hours at night. It is no surprise, then, that normal people with "normal" spines wake up with some back or neck stiffness after a good night's sleep and no surprise that some people with back, neck or other joint or muscle problems wake up stiffer and need some time or a hot shower to get going in the morning.

When viewed from the side, the spine is not straight (Fig. 2-8, Fig. 1-2). Therefore, it is hard to imagine that sleeping on a rigid, flat surface could be comfortable or beneficial for your spine. Rather, a surface that gives support, yet conforms to your body shape and also distributes that support, should be a lot more comfortable and beneficial for your spine.

It is difficult and impossible to say with certainty that any single or specific sleeping surface is the best for everyone. Some say that a hard floor is the best sleeping surface for people with or without back or neck pain; others say that soft or firm mattresses are best; others that waterbeds are best. Recommendations for pillows range from none to one to many and the shape, contour and softness or firmness recommendations are just as variable.

Hopefully everyone can figure out for themselves what is the best mattress and pillow for them but unfortunately, many of us are still looking. We (the authors) do not and will not say that any one sleeping method or surface is guaranteed the best. It certainly makes sense that a mattress or pillow that conforms to the shape of the spine and supports, but distributes uniformly the pressures on the spine and different body parts would be ideal. For these reasons, we have been very impressed with the Tempur-Pedic products and would encourage you to read Chapter 5.

OTHER CAUSES OF BACK AND NECK PAIN

Although the main causes of back and neck pain are traumatic, degenerative or idiopathic in origin, a number of other factors or conditions may also cause pain. For simplicity's sake, we have grouped them under the title "other causes." These other causes occur less frequently than traumatic, degenerative or idiopathic pain and are significantly different in origin. Included in this category are developmental pain, inflammatory pain, pain from infection, pain from neoplasm (tumor) and metabolic pain.

Developmental Pain

The fetal development of the spine and its components is quite complex. Congenital abnormalities of the spine vary from insignificant problems to major defects in the spinal bones or spinal cord and nerves. Abnormalities that develop with growth can likewise vary from mild to severe. They may be associated with no pain, or they may be the cause of disabling back or neck pain.

As the spine grows and develops, especially during the growth spurts of childhood and adolescence, problems can occur. As mentioned, the spine viewed from behind is straight and when viewed from the side has a lazy S curve to it. When viewing the spine from the side, kyphosis or round back is an increased angulation in the mid-thoracic spine, whereas lordosis is an increased angulation of the lower spine (Figure 2-8). Scoliosis is a lateral or "sideways" curvature of the spine as seen when it is viewed from behind (Figure 2-9). These conditions may have no discernible cause (idiopathic), or there may be a localized or generalized growth abnormality.

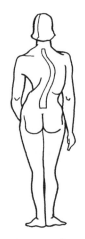

Figure 2-9   Scoliosis (curvature of the spine)

An example of a localized developmental abnormality is spondylolysis, which is a defect in the bony architecture of the lumbar spine that may allow forward slipping (spondylolisthesis) of one vertebrae on another (Figure 2-10). This condition can lead to an increase in lumbar lordosis and, if it is severe enough, can result in pinching of the spinal cord and nerves. Spondylolisthesis can be caused by a fracture in the spine, but more often it is an unrecognized, not completely understood, developmental process that occurs in the growing child.

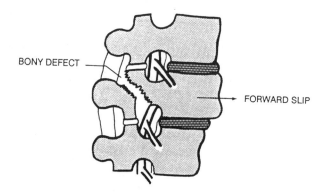

BONY DEFECT

FORWARD SLIP

Figure 2-10   Spondylolysis and spondylolisthesis

Inflammatory Pain

The word arthritis means inflammation of a joint. Osteoarthritis refers to the degenerative arthritis that occurs as part of the normal aging process or following an injury. Inflammatory arthritis refers to those conditions such as rheumatoid arthritis and ankylosing spondylitis that can affect the joints of the body, including the spine (Figure 2-11).

Inflammation occurs in all arthritis. In osteoarthritis, the inflammation is secondary to the degenerative process. In inflammatory arthritis, the inflammation itself is the primary process and the cause of pain or dysfunction.

The pain of inflammatory arthritis is often similar to degenerative pain in that it comes on slowly and progressively, but there is no history of a significant injury. In addition, inflammatory arthritis usually occurs at an earlier age and is often associated with inflammatory joint problems. Conditions such as rheumatoid arthritis and ankylosing spondylitis can be detected with blood tests.

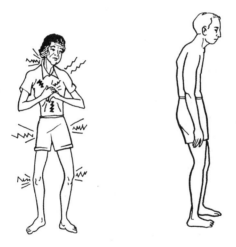

Figure 2-11   Inflammatory spine pain: rheumatoid arthritis (left) and ankylosing spondylitis (right)

Pain From Infection

Infection is a rare cause of back and neck pain and can involve the bones (vertebrae), the discs or the spinal cord (meningitis). Infection can spread from other parts of the body through the bloodstream to the spine. In children, spinal infections usually follow respiratory tract infections. In adults, spinal infections may follow kidney or urinary tract infections. Infections can also occur after spinal surgery.

Pain From Neoplasm (Tumor)

Abnormal tumors or growths—cancerous or noncancerous—can involve your spine and any of its components and cause pain. These growths can originate in your spine or spread to your spine from a cancerous tumor elsewhere in your body.

Metabolic Pain

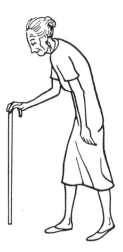

Metabolic causes of back and neck pain are those that result in abnormal or insufficient bone. A common metabolic cause of back pain is osteoporosis. Osteoporosis is a decrease in the mineral substance of bone that results in a weakening of the bone. It occurs most commonly in elderly people, especially post-menopausal women. This process, to a certain extent, normally

Figure 2-12
Metabolic back pain

occurs later in life, but may be accelerated by a combination of hormonal and dietary factors, as well as decreased physical activity. Osteoporosis can be a source of back pain and can also result in vertebral compression fractures. Many other metabolic diseases can cause problems in bone formation, including scurvy, rickets, kidney dysfunction and other hormonal imbalances.

THE NEXT STEP

In our opinion, understanding the cause of your back and neck pain is more important than understanding the specific anatomical structure involved. Once you are aware of the cause of your pain, it is easier to then understand which anatomical structure is involved. The basic causes of back pain were examined in abbreviated detail in this chapter. Keep in mind that the list of potential causes of back and neck pain is almost endless. We've attempted to provide you with an overview of the most common conditions.

In the next chapter, the evaluation process used by physicians to diagnose and evaluate the specific causes of back or neck pain is described, including the typical history and the type of pain associated with each cause of back or neck pain.

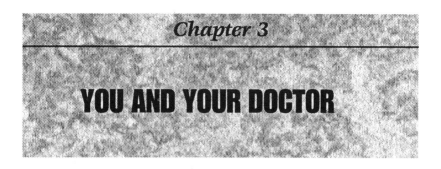

Chapter 3

YOU AND YOUR DOCTOR

"Pain is oft a visitant; but pain clings cruelly to us."
—John Keats

If your back or neck pain shows signs of being more than a minor problem, you should see a doctor. For example, if you have persistent pain down one of your arms or legs, it can be more than a minor problem. Your back or neck pain can also be serious if it is accompanied by other symptoms, such as weakness in one of your arms or legs, or bowel or bladder dysfunction. This chapter presents guidelines on selecting a doctor to diagnose and treat your back or neck pain. Also included is an abbreviated overview of the process used by physicians to evaluate your back or neck pain. Finally, suggestions on whether or not you should seek out a second medical opinion on your back or neck pain are presented.

SELECTING A DOCTOR

As a rule, your choice of a physician to treat your back or neck pain will be between a general practice doctor, an orthopedic specialist, a neurosurgeon or neurologist and an osteopath. Many individuals also choose either a physical therapist or a chiropractor to attend to their back or neck pain.

A general practice or family practice doctor is trained to deal with a wide variety of medical problems and patients of all ages. General practitioners are also sources of referrals for patients requiring specialized treatment. Orthopedic specialists are individuals who specialize in bone and joint problems and whose training involves attention to the mechanical, structural and architectural factors relating to your spine. Neurologists and neurosurgeons are specialists in the central and peripheral nervous systems. Osteopaths undergo training generally equivalent to an M.D.'s but with an emphasis on spinal manipulation. Physical therapists are registered health-care technologists who specialize in rehabilitative exercise. Chiropractors are licensed health-care specialists who utilize spinal manipulation as their primary means of therapy.

Not surprisingly, no hard-and-fast rule exists that you can apply to the task of selecting your doctor. Your primary selection criteria must be that the doctor is eminently qualified to make an accurate assessment of your problem and capable of administering the appropriate treatment therapy. The trained specialist you select to treat your spine should treat backs and necks on a regular basis and should be thoroughly up to date on the most current information and techniques for treating back and neck pain.

Whereas a physician's reputation and the recommendation of someone whose opinion you respect can guide you to your initial choice of a doctor, you still need to use your own judgment. Knowing as much as possible about how your spine works and what the general causes of back and neck pain are can help you proceed more reasonably. A basic understanding of how your doctor will diagnose and evaluate your back or neck pain is invaluable. The more you understand the entire process, including how your spine functions and the disorders that impair these functions and cause pain, the better you will be able to decide whether or not your doctor is treating you in a satisfactory manner.

EVALUATING AND DIAGNOSING YOUR BACK AND NECK PAIN

Having identified the person you would like to serve as your doctor, the next step is to undergo a thorough evaluation. When physicians or health care specialists are evaluating any musculoskeletal problem, be it a knee, ankle, shoulder, back or neck injury, their thought processes are basically the same. First a history of the problem is obtained, then a physical examination is performed and finally special studies such as X-rays are ordered. Each of these three aspects of this investigative effort is important in the overall evaluation of back or neck pain and any other musculoskeletal problem (Figure 3-1). The more thorough the analysis of all aspects of your back problem, the more effective your doctor will be in prescribing proper treatment.

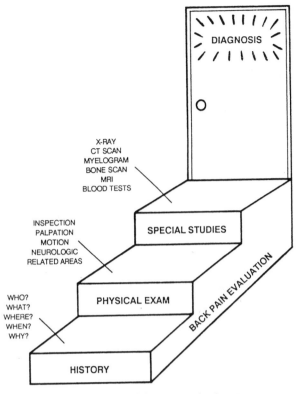

Figure 3-1   Evaluating and diagnosing back pain

HISTORY

Obtaining a good history from patients about their problems is probably the most important information in the overall investigative process because it is the first step in the evaluation of back or neck pain. Obtaining a history may be simple, or it may require some detective work, but it should at least start off with some very simple information. A history usually involves having the patient complete a written questionnaire. A good history answers the questions: who, what, where, when, and why. Table 3-1 presents the histories of three people experiencing back pain:

1. A 16-year-old female gymnast who fell yesterday at practice and now has sharp pain in her lower back.
2. A 70-year-old retired accountant who has had dull pain in his low back for 20 years, but can't remember any injury.
3. A 30-year-old healthy recreational athlete who has experienced sharp and dull low back pain off and on for several years but can't recall any injury.

WHO? (patient information)	WHAT? (type of pain)	WHERE? (location of pain)	WHEN? (onset of pain)	WHY? (cause of pain)
16-year-old female gymnast	sharp pain	low back	yesterday	injury (traumatic)
70-year-old retired accountant	dull pain	low back	20 years ago	wear and tear (degenerative)
30-year-old healthy recreational athlete	sharp and dull pain	low back	several years ago	??? (idiopathic)

Table 3-1   Three patient histories

Each of these three people has low back pain, but their stories are significantly different. In each case, a thorough history (answering the simple questions who, what, where, when and why) makes it easy to see why their stories are different. A good history is the starting point in the evaluation process of their back pain and can even allow us to make some presumptions about the cause of their back pain.

The terms discussed in Chapter 2 that describe the causes of back pain are: 1) traumatic, 2) degenerative, and 3) idiopathic. It is easy to categorize each of these three patients into a presumptive category of back pain according to the cause of the pain:

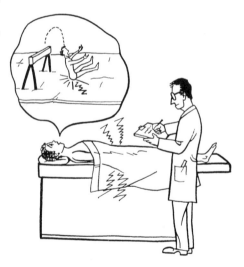

1) The 16-year-old gymnast has traumatic back pain (Figure 3-2).
2) The 70-year-old retired accountant has degenerative back pain (Figure 3-3).
3) The 30-year-old healthy recreational athlete has idiopathic back pain (Figure 3-4).

Figure 3-2

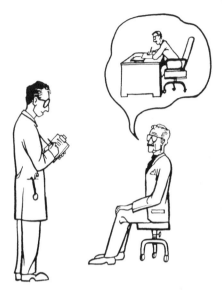

Figure 3-3

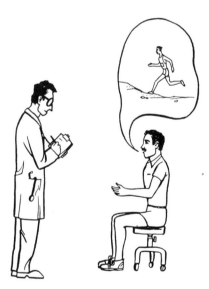

Figure 3-4

In addition to the cause of the pain, it is important to further investigate the type of pain, because this also can be a clue to the origin of the pain. Although it may be difficult to categorize types of pain precisely, there are three basic types of pain that occur in your back.

Type 1 pain can be fairly well localized and originates in the superficial structures (skin, spinous processes, interspinal ligaments and spinal muscles). This is the type of pain seen in acute traumatic back pain and is the type of pain that the 16-year-old gymnast is having.

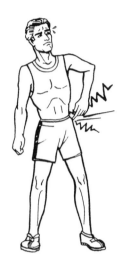

Figure 3-5   Type 1 pain

Type 2 pain is a deep, aching pain, not as well localized as Type 1 pain. It is usually the result of problems in the bony framework of the spine (the vertebrae, facet joints and discs). This pain may radiate into the flanks or buttocks. This is the type of pain seen in chronic traumatic, degenerative or idiopathic back pain and is the type of pain both the 70-year-old accountant and the 30-year-old recreational athlete are having.

Type 3 pain is caused by irritation of the spinal nerves and is intense, sharp and electric in nature. The degree of pain depends on

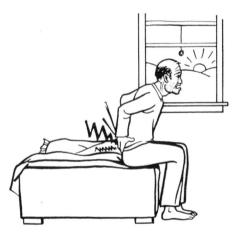

Figure 3-6   Type 2 pain

the amount of nerve compression and can cause back pain that shoots into the lower leg or neurologic changes such as a decrease in sensation and strength in the lower leg. This is the type of pain present in sciatica.

Obviously, these pain patterns overlap and may occur together if there is a combination of problems.

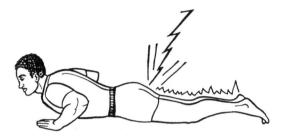

Figure 3-7   Type 3 pain

PHYSICAL EXAMINATION

Just as obtaining a history starts off simple and becomes more complex, the physical examination does as well. An organized physical examination proceeds in a step-by-step fashion and consists of the following: (Figure 3-8):

1. General inspection
2. Palpation (feeling)
3. Measuring motion
4. Neurologic examination
5. Examination of related areas

General Inspection

A great deal of information can be obtained by merely looking at someone and watching him or her move about. It doesn't take a medically trained eye to tell the difference between a person who is obviously out of shape, over-

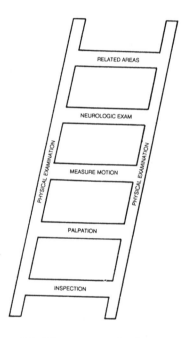

Figure 3-8   The components of a physical examination

weight and has poor posture and a person who is fit and trim with good posture (Figure 3-9). Likewise, if you have ever had or know someone who has had a severe case of low back pain, you know it is obvious to everyone around that something is wrong.

During the physical examination, the doctor inspects your spine both from the side and back while you stand. Since the spine should have a lazy S curve to it when viewed from the side, one of the first things your doctor looks for is an increase or decrease in these curves. Individuals with a spasm in their back muscles may have a straight, stiff spine, whereas a pregnant woman would likely have an increased curve in her lower back caused by her additional abdominal weight.

Viewed from the back, your spine should appear straight. Your shoulders and hips should also be level, balanced, and symmetric in appearance. If they are not, the spine may be curved (scoliosis). Your doctor should also measure each of your legs because a difference in their lengths may also account for an

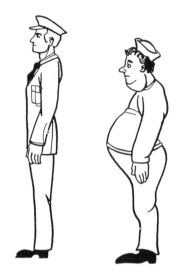

Figure 3-9   "General Inspection"

imbalance in the hip or shoulder area. A doctor examining the areas surrounding your spine will also be able to tell whether or not you have any obvious deformity or swelling, skin abnormalities or muscle atrophy.

Palpation

After a general inspection is performed, a doctor will palpate the bones, muscles and soft tissues of your spine to feel for tenderness, spasm and deformity. The spinous processes (bony prominences of the posterior aspect of the spine), as well as the interspinous ligaments between each spinous process, should be examined from your skull to your pelvis. Your doctor should feel for deformity and determine the precise areas that are painful to touch. The bones of your pelvis are also palpated. Your paraspinal, gluteal, thigh and abdominal muscles will also be examined for pain and spasm.

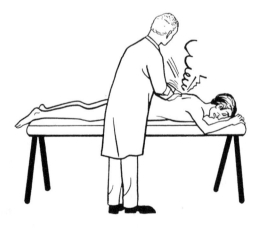

Figure 3-10   Palpation

Range of Motion

Your spine can move in a number of directions. Measuring the motion of your spine to determine if you are restricted in motion or if a certain motion is painful is another step in the physical examination of your spine. The movements of the spine are flexion, extension, lateral bending and rotation. To test flexion, you are required to bend over with your knees straight to see how close you can get your fingertips to the ground. Extension is bending backwards. Lateral bending and rotation should be comparable going each way (Figure 3-11). These motion tests are performed to evaluate any significant restriction in spinal motion.

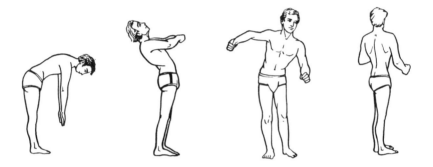

Figure 3-11 Determining range of motion (left to right): flexion, extension, lateral bending, and rotation

Dysfunction of any of the components of your spine can cause painful or restricted motion. A problem with the bones or ligaments of your spine, muscle tightness or spasm, or sciatic nerve irritation can all affect the amount of motion of your spine.

The straight leg raise test (Figure 3-12) is one of the motion tests commonly used by physicians to evaluate your low back. To perform the straight leg raise test, begin by lying flat on your back. Keeping your legs straight, your doctor raises one of them into the air and measures the angle that your leg can be raised from the horizontal. A normal straight leg raise is 90 degrees or more.

The motion measured by the straight leg raise test can be limited by a number of factors, including pain in your back, tightness in your hamstring muscles and irritation of your sciatic nerve. It is important to try to determine the limiting factor in performing this straight leg raise. If the restricting factor involves your back, low back pain will occur with the maneuver. If it is tight hamstrings, pain or tightness will be felt in the back of your upper leg or behind your knee when the test is performed. If the limiting factor is an irritated

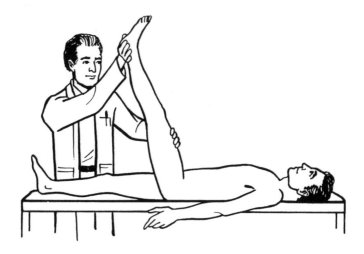

Figure 3-12   The straight leg raise test

sciatic nerve, you will experience shooting pains into the involved leg because the straight leg raise test puts tension on that nerve.

Neurological Examination

In the lumbar spine (lower back), the sciatic nerve is a combination of several spinal nerves that exit the spinal column independently, merge into one large nerve and descend to the lower leg through your buttocks and thigh all the way to your foot (Figure 3-13). When your sciatic nerve is irritated, there may be tenderness along the course of the nerve. The area that the sciatic nerve travels through in the buttocks (the sciatic notch) can be palpated deep in the buttock between two

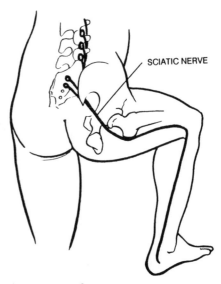

Figure 3-13   The sciatic nerve

bony prominences, one on your hip and the other on your pelvis. If your sciatic nerve is irritated (sciatica), then palpation of the sciatic notch will be painful. Also, if sciatica is present, the straight leg raise test will cause shooting pains along the course of the nerve into your foot because performing the test increases tension and pressure on the already irritated sciatic nerve.

Your doctor will also check your sciatic nerve by assessing the sensation, muscle function and reflexes in your leg. Additionally, the several spinal nerves that combined to form the sciatic nerve should each be individually tested. The three spinal nerves most affected in sciatica are the fourth lumbar (L4), fifth lumbar (L5), and first sacral (S1) nerves.

The L4 nerve exits your spine at the level of fourth lumbar vertebra, supplies sensation to the inside of your foot and is mainly responsible for the muscle that raises your ankle (anterior tibial muscle). It is also responsible for the knee jerk reflex.

The L5 nerve exits at the fifth lumbar vertebra, supplies sensation to the top of your foot and works the muscle that raises your big toe (extensor hallucis longus muscle).

The S1 nerve exits at the first sacral vertebra, supplies sensation to the outside of your foot, works the muscles that allow your ankle and foot to move downward (gastrocnemius and soleus muscles) and controls the ankle jerk reflex.

In the cervical spine (neck), there are a number of nerves that exit the spinal column and go to the shoulder or through the axilla (armpit) to various parts of the arm and hand. When these nerves are irritated, there may be tenderness along the course of the nerve. Bending or twisting your neck or putting pressure on the top of your head can increase the pressure on a cervical spine nerve and cause more pain.

Just as with the sciatic nerve, your doctor will examine your cervical nerves by assessing the sensation and muscle function in your shoulder, arm and hand.

The C5 nerve exits at the level of the fifth cervical vertebra, supplies sensation to the upper arm and is mainly responsible for the shoulder muscles.

The C6 nerve exits at the sixth cervical vertebra, supplies sensation to the forearm, thumb and index finger and is mainly responsible for the muscles that allow you to extend your wrist.

The C7 nerve exits at the seventh cervical vertebra, supplies sensation to the middle finger and is mainly responsible for the muscles that allow you to flex your wrist and extend your fingers.

The C8 nerve is interestingly named, because there is no eighth cervical vertebra. The C8 nerve exits between the seventh cervical vertebra and the first thoracic vertebra. It supplies sensation to the ring and little fingers and is mainly responsible for the muscles that allow you to flex your fingers.

Obviously, in the arms, hands and legs, there is overlap in which nerve root is responsible for working the different muscles. However, your doctor, with a good physical exam, should be able to figure out which nerve is irritated or not working correctly.

Examination of Related Areas

Although this book is concerned with back and neck pain caused by problems in your spine, you should remember that other areas of your body can refer pain to your back and may also need to be examined. Painful conditions, such as hip arthritis, may initially mimic back pain. Problems in your hips, knees or ankles can also affect your spine and cause back pain. In addition, stomach, intestinal, kidney, pelvis and other internal problems may manifest themselves as back pain (Figure 3-14).

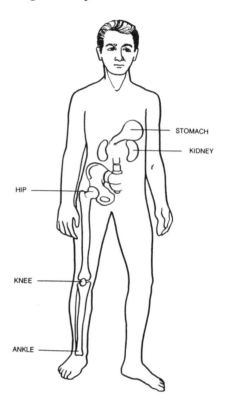

Figure 3-14   Examination of related areas

X-Rays and other Studies

After completion of a history and a physical examination, your doctor may decide that it is appropriate to order X-rays and other studies to assist in an evaluation of your back or neck pain. Regular X-rays are usually the initial test used to evaluate the bones of your spine, just as they are used to evaluate the bones elsewhere in your body. Other X-ray studies, such as a computerized tomography (CT scan), magnetic resonance imaging (MRI), myelogram, or bone scan, are also sometimes used in an evaluation of back or neck pain. Blood work is occasionally another component of the evaluative process for back or neck pain. All of these tests, however, should complement—not replace—the history of your back or neck pain and a thorough physical examination.

Depending on the history of your back or neck pain and the results of your physical examination, your doctor may decide that it is not appropriate to order X-rays for you. On the other hand, your history and physical examination may indicate that extensive testing is required. The process and relative need for testing is illustrated by the following two examples:

1. A 10-year-old active boy falls off his slow-moving bike but continues to play all day and only complains the next day to his mother that he has a little pain in his back. At this time, it is probably not worth exposing this young boy to the unnecessary radiation of X-rays.

2. A previously healthy 20-year-old athlete injured her back two weeks ago and now has progressive pain in her back and legs with numbness and weakness in her legs. In this instance, extensive testing to determine the cause of this problem could be indicated.

X-Rays

Regular X-rays are usually the initial study ordered in an evaluation of back or neck problems. Most always, a minimum of two X-rays are obtained. One is a front-to-back view of your spine, and the other is a side view. Other X-ray views, such as oblique views, may also be taken to get a different view of the bones of your spine. X-rays of your spine will show if there is a problem with the bones of your spine, such as a fracture, arthritis, bone spurs or a curvature of the spine (Figure 3-15).

Computerized Tomography (CT) Scan

A CT scan is a special X-ray study that adds a three-dimensional effect to an X-ray evaluation of your spine (Figure 3-16). A CT scan provides your physician with a cross sectional view of your spine, rather than the front-to-back, side or oblique views produced by regular X-rays. The cross sectional view seen on a CT scan is the view you would have if you were able to see your spine from above. The level of your spine that is to be evaluated by a CT scan can be varied so that multiple cross sectional views are obtained.

A CT scan shows not only the bones of your spine, but also the soft tissues, such as the discs, the spinal cord and the nerves. A CT scan may be used in the evaluation of the bones of your spine because it provides a view different than regular X-rays, and therefore can be helpful in assessing fractures or arthritis. Because it gives multiple cross sectional views of your spine and the area that your spinal cord occupies, a CT scan is very helpful in determining if there is pressure on your spinal cord or nerves from an injured disc or from arthritis. A CT scan has about five times the radiation than that of a regular X-ray study of the spine.

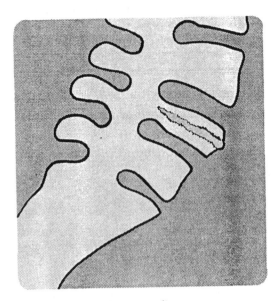

*Figure 3-15   An X-ray revealing a
compression fracture*

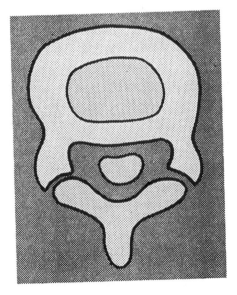

Figure 3-16   CT scan

Magnetic Resonance Imaging (MRI)

MRI is the most recently developed of the various types of studies used in the evaluation of the spine. The images created by MRI are made using magnetic fields that do not produce radiation exposure. MRI combines the benefits of regular x-rays and CT scans to provide a picture that shows not only the bones, but also the soft tissues (Figure 3-17). Accordingly, MRI results can be very valuable in helping to evaluate the structures of your back, especially pressure on your spinal cord from a disc injury, arthritis or bone spurs.

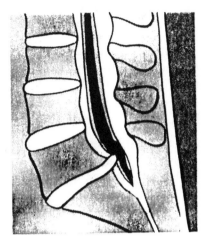

Figure 3-17   Magnetic resonance imaging showing a herniated disc.

Bone Scan

A bone scan (Figure 3-18) is a study performed by injecting a radioactive labeled material into your bloodstream and then using a machine like a Geiger counter to measure the amount of this material absorbed in your bones. The material that is injected contains phosphorous, which is one of the minerals normally found in bone. When phosphorous is injected into your bloodstream, it is absorbed into the bone in small amounts. By adding a small amount of non-danger-

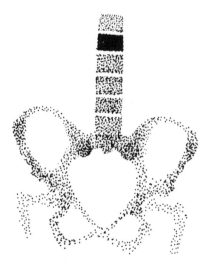

Figure 3-18   Bone scan showing increased activity in L1 vertebra

ous radioactive phosphorous to this solution, the phosphorous that is taken up by the bones can then be measured by the Geiger counter. If there is an area in which bone is actively being made, such as a recent fracture that is healing, uptake of the phosphorous solution by that bone is much greater than in the surrounding bones. This process is shown by increased activity or uptake on the bone scan. In addition to a fracture, other bone processes that make or destroy bone will usually be apparent on a bone scan. Fractures, infections and arthritis will increase bone activity, whereas tumors may either increase or decrease activity.

Although bone scans do not provide the detail of regular X-rays, they do give a different type of information that may be valuable in the evaluation of back pain. A bone scan has about five times the radiation of a regular X-ray study of the spine.

Myelogram

A myelogram is an X-ray study done after a special dye is injected into the fluid surrounding your spinal cord and nerves (Figure 3-19). After the dye is injected into the spinal fluid, regular X-rays or a CT scan can be performed.

Normally the spinal fluid flows freely around the spinal cord up and down your spine from your brain (above) to your lower back (below). If pressure exists on your spinal cord or nerves, the spinal fluid will not flow freely. An X-ray taken after an injection of the

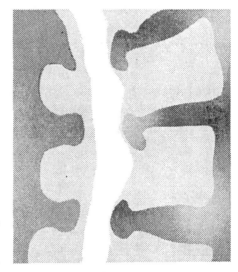

Figure 3-19   Myelogram

dye will show an indentation on the spinal cord or nerves. A disc that has slipped, ruptured or herniated will cause pressure on the spinal cord and produce an indentation that can be seen on a myelogram study. The same thing can happen if there is a displaced fracture, a bone spur or a significant arthritis of the bones of your spine.

Blood Tests

In the evaluation of back and neck pain, it may also be appropriate to order blood or other laboratory tests. Blood tests can show if an inflammatory arthritis, such as rheumatoid arthritis or ankylosing spondylitis, is present. Blood tests can also help indicate whether or not an infection is present. Blood or other laboratory tests can also provide valuable information to enable your doctor to determine if other problems, such as tumors or kidney infections, may be causing your back or neck pain.

GETTING A SECOND OPINION

"Get a second opinion" is advice that is often easier given than acted upon. Whether or not you decide to pursue this course of action is entirely up to you. Whether or not you should feel the need to consider getting a second opinion depends on any number of factors. Do you have confidence in your doctor? Would a second opinion enhance your confidence in your doctor's advice? What are the risk factors involved in your doctor's advice? Obviously, the greater the risks, the greater your need to do all you can to make sure that you select the best course of action. And remember, the choice is yours and yours alone. Do you feel like you've been rushed into considering surgery by your doctor? Have you had a previous operation for the same condition? Has your doctor guaranteed the results from the proposed surgery? Has your doctor explained your situation to you in terms that you can understand? Do you believe you've been treated fairly?

If you decide to obtain a second opinion, it should be from a doctor who is at least as well qualified as the first. Once you've opted for a second opinion, however, you must decide what to do if the second opinion differs substantially from the first. We strongly recommend that you remember that you should not permit yourself to be rushed into a decision on what treatment you should adopt. Only in rare instances (paralysis or increasing loss of sensation or motor power) is time a crucial factor in your decision. So proceed cautiously —don't make a hasty decision.

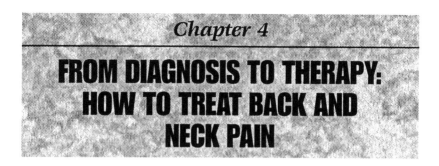

Chapter 4

FROM DIAGNOSIS TO THERAPY: HOW TO TREAT BACK AND NECK PAIN

"Primum non nocere." (First of all, do no harm.)
—Hippocrates

The statistics on back and neck pain present an extraordinarily bleak picture: over 10 million sufferers annually, over 100 million workdays lost every year, over 5 billion dollars in direct and indirect treatment costs and bouts of pain and intolerable anguish so seemingly countless as to give new meaning to the term "implausible." And yet, for all of the world's technological advances, for all of the evolutionary advances in the body of medical knowledge relating to pain, a simple fact remains: the mysteries of back pain often defy simple solutions. It is somewhat easier to explain why this is so than to accept the explanation. At best, medicine is not an exact science. If it were, surely a world in which the means were created for travel among the stars of the outer reaches of the universe would find a way to identify a foolproof method of treating (and preventing) back and neck pain.

Since you have purchased this book and are reading this chapter, we assume that you have painfully discovered that considerable debate exists within the medical community on how to effectively treat back and neck pain. This chapter presents an overview of the most typical approaches and means for treating back and neck pain. For discussion purposes, the possible therapies are divided into two groups: nonsurgical and surgical.

NONSURGICAL THERAPIES

First, the good news. The natural course of back and neck pain is that it will go away with time. Your chances of not needing surgery to treat your back or neck condition are excellent. Most pain can be eliminated by letting nature take its course and giving it time to go away or through one or a combination of any of the nonsurgical therapies discussed in this section. In fact, the need for much of the surgery currently conducted has been subject to considerable questioning. Now, the bad news. There are no guarantees—no treatment, surgical or nonsurgical, can guarantee elimination of your pain.

Physicians have found that most of the nonsurgical therapies discussed in this section have a 60 to 70 percent chance of being successful. Which one should you use? This is something that you should discuss with your doctor. In fact, were you to check with several different physicians, it is likely that you would receive several different pieces of advice. Our advice to you is to try two or three of the nonsurgical treatment options. If your pain persists after your nonsurgical efforts, it is then time to consider other alternatives.

Bed Rest

Lying in bed (except for an occasional visit to the bathroom) is the most commonly prescribed treatment for back and neck pain, particularly in the acute phase. Bed rest is frequently effective because it reduces the mechanical irritation of your spine and diminishes the level of inflammation in the area surrounding the irritation. As a result, this may enable you to become pain-free without any additional action on your part. There are at least two possible problems, however, with bed rest therapy. First, it doesn't work for everyone. In fact some individuals find that their back or neck pain is aggravated by lying down. Second, most individuals don't have the time or patience to spend two to three days or weeks in bed. All too clearly, they realize that whatever factor initially caused their pain is likely to do so again in the not too distant future. Despite these potential problems, bed rest is the oldest, and possibly the most widely prescribed, therapy for treating back and neck pain. (Note: Detailed guidelines for the most appropriate position for lying in bed for preventing back and neck pain are presented in Chapter 6.)

Drug Therapy

Drugs and medicines are commonly used in the treatment of back and neck pain. They generally fall into three categories: (1) painkillers, (2) anti-inflammatory medicines and (3) muscle relaxants.

Historically, the most widely used drug has been aspirin. Aspirin is both a mild painkiller and an anti-inflammatory medicine. It will relieve the pain of an injury or chronic condition and also help relieve the inflammation that causes the pain, thereby serving a dual purpose. It is available without a prescription, inexpensive and reasonably safe. Anyone with bleeding tendencies or gastrointestinal problems needs to be careful taking aspirin and other anti-inflammatory medicines. Tylenol is another commonly used non-prescription mild pain relieving medicine. Tylenol, however, is not an anti-inflammatory medicine and therefore probably will not do as well as aspirin or other anti-inflammatory medicines when a component of the pain problem is inflammation.

Anti-inflammatory medicines (other than aspirin) are now available without a prescription and include Ibuprofen (Advil, Motrin, Datril), Aleve and Orudis-KT. Prescription anti-inflammatory medicines are very numerous (and usually more expensive) and include Anaprox, Ansaid, Cataflam, Clinoril, Daypro, Dolobid, Feldene, Indocin, Lodine, Motrin, Nalfon, Naprosyn, Orudis, Oruvail, Relafen, Tolectin, Toradol and Voltaren.

Anti-inflammatory medicines work because they relieve or stop the inflammation that is causing your pain. Although all anti-inflammatory medicines work in a similar fashion, they are different, so if one doesn't work, you can try another one. We recommend using the anti-inflammatory medicine, either prescription or non prescription that is the best tolerated by your system, inexpensive and works for you. If you need to take an anti-inflammatory medicine for an ongoing problem, we recommend taking it, as directed, for 5-7 days to give it a chance to work. If you develop problems, you should obviously stop the medicine and consult your physician. You should not be taking more than one type of anti-inflammatory medicine at a time. If you have to take anti-inflammatory medicines for a prolonged period of time you should do so under the guidance of your physician.

Prescription painkillers include pills and shots: Codeine (Tylenol #3), Darvocet, Darvon, Demerol, Dilaudid, Hydrocodone (Lorcet, Lortab, Vicodin), Oxycodone (Percocet, Percodan, Tylox), Talwin and Ultram.

Prescription pain medicines can cause constipation, drowsiness, nausea, light-headedness and can be addicting. You should not be driving a car or working around heavy or dangerous equipment when taking prescription pain medicines. The elderly need to be especially cautious with this type of medicine.

Muscle relaxants are also sometimes prescribed for the treatment of back or neck pain. If a stiff muscle is the source of your pain and preventing you from relaxing or resting, a muscle relaxant may

benefit you. Some of the more commonly prescribed muscle relaxants include Flexeril, Norflex, Norgesic, Parafon Forte, Robaxin, Soma
and Valium. The same precautions taken for prescription pain medicines apply to muscle relaxants.

Just as with anti-inflammatory medicines, if you are having
trouble taking a prescription pain medicine or muscle relaxant, you
should stop taking the medicine and consult your physician. There is
minimal risk in taking any of these medicines for a short period of
time and usually minimal risk of taking medicines for a long period
of time that you can buy without a prescription. The risks of taking
prescription anti-inflammatory medicines for a prolonged period of
time are also minimal but should be done under the guidance of your
physician. Taking prescription painkiller medicine and muscle relaxants for any length of time is obviously risky.

Spinal Manipulation

This method involves manipulating the spine, ostensibly to realign the joints of the spine, with particular attention given to the
condition of the soft tissues of the back and neck and to the level of
muscle relaxation. In general, most manipulations are indirectly performed on the pain sufferer. The sufferer's head, shoulders and hips
are twisted by someone in an attempt to realign the spine. Direct
manipulation is conducted by applying pressure directly to the spinous
processes of specific vertebrae.

The most common practitioners of spinal manipulation are chiropractors. All factors considered, they generally enjoy wide popularity. Osteopathic physicians also regularly employ manipulation as a
treatment therapy for back and neck pain. In addition to spinal manipulation, chiropractors and osteopathic physicians typically utilize
many of the other nonsurgical therapies discussed on the following
pages.

With regard to spinal manipulation, two questions arise: "Does
it work?" and "What are the dangers attendant to manipulation?" The
answer to the first question depends almost entirely on who you ask.
There is obviously a lot of positive subjective opinion among many of
the individuals who have undergone manipulation, or it wouldn't be
as popular as it is. On the other hand, argue critics of this technique,
there is no statistical evidence to support the claim that spinal manipulation produces a greater reduction in back pain than nature's
own healing. In view of the potential dangers, however slight, these
individuals conclude that the potential risks of spinal manipulation
outweigh the possible gains. The primary risk is the danger that "jos-
tling" the spine, discs and nerves can result in worsening your condition or cause a far more serious injury. However rare the risks, some

individuals would prefer to wait for nature to take its course. Others prefer to try out their options as soon as possible. It is hoped that research which is currently being conducted on spinal manipulation therapy will provide more definitive information in the future about its usefulness.

Heat/Cold Therapy

Applying heat or cold to the area of your spine that is painful (using an ice pack, heating pad or lamp) is one of the oldest and most useful methods for relieving muscle spasms. Neither heat nor cold has any curative effects, but each is often successful in relieving muscle spasms. Although heat and cold are opposites, they accomplish the same thing in treating back pain—they increase blood flow to the affected area. Heat involves a reflex mechanism that stimulates the attendant nerves. In turn, the blood vessels in the area to which heat is applied become dilated (expanded) so that more blood flows and the metabolism of the muscles in the area (including the one that is in spasm) is increased. The net result is that spasm "relaxes."

Applying cold to the area is also effective. Whereas heat expands the blood vessels, cold constricts them. Cold is used following an acute injury to minimize bleeding in an injured area and to minimize swelling. And yet, after cold is used for a period of time, the constricted blood vessels fatigue, and then they relax and dilate. In the end, then, cold and heat have essentially the same effect. Because it is more comfortable, most people prefer heat to cold. In reality, though, cold is uncomfortable only for the first few minutes. Then the area becomes numb. A momentary burning sensation is usually experienced when cold is first applied, but it subsides quickly as the cold therapy is continued.

Two basic questions arise concerning the use of heat or cold as a therapy for treating back pain: "In what form should either be applied?" and "How often should the therapy be used?" Heat can be used in many forms. The simplest, least expensive ones have been found to be as effective as the more expensive methods. At home, you can use a hot water bottle, a heating pad or a water-heated towel to provide the heat. In general, wet heat has been found to be more successful for most people than dry heat. Wet or dry, you should apply the heat to your muscle spasm for approximately 20 to 30 minutes each session, two to four times a day. If you are particularly fortunate or resourceful, a hot tub is often an effective method for relieving a muscle spasm. Physicians will sometimes use deep heat as part of their treatment efforts for your back. Usually these efforts involve either diathermy or ultrasound. Diathermy uses a machine which, when applied to the area, produces a rapidly alternating electrical field that produces heat below the surface area of your skin by inducing movement in the molecules of your body's tissues. Ultrasound is the deepest form of heat therapy. The ultrasound waves, when applied to your skin where your pain is located, vibrate deep in your tissues, agitating the molecules in the tissues, and in turn causing them to produce heat in the affected area.

Cold is usually applied using an ice pack. Like heat, cold should be used two to four times a day. Ice packs should be applied to the affected area for 15 to 20 minutes at a time. A more effective way to use ice for cold therapy is to massage or rub the ice over the affected area. A technique that can be used for doing this is to freeze paper cups three-quarters filled with water. Then simply tear away just enough of the top portion of the cup to expose the ice and gently rub the skin over the affected area with it. Ice should be applied for approximately 30 seconds longer once the area being rubbed feels numb.

Massage

Like heat/cold therapy, massage is a method for treating muscle spasms that involves no risks and often provides immediate relief. Massage is passive exercise. Most massage treatments are applied painlessly by having someone rub or knead selected areas of your body. For most individuals, the process has psychological, as well as physiological, benefits. Psychologically, the stroking of our bodies has a soothing effect. Physiologically, massage stimulates the nervous system, which in turn elicits a response by your respiratory and circulatory systems. More blood is brought to the muscle in spasm because the blood vessels are dilated. Nourishment is delivered via the blood to the affected area, and more waste products are removed. The (desired) net result is that massage helps to relax muscles in spasm. Specific types of massage include home (nonprofessional) massage, professional massage, connective tissue massage and zone therapy. Although none of these forms has any documented curative powers, each seems to be an effective means of relieving back pain for some people.

Back/Neck Support Devices

A wide variety of braces, corsets and collars is currently on the market. Collectively, these devices purport to help relieve back pain by providing abdominal support and relieve back or neck pain by supporting the spine. The better planned back devices are designed for effective abdominal compression and for a slightly flexed lumbar spine. Lumbar flexion minimizes the degree to which the lumbar disc can bulge backwards, and it decreases some of the forces on the lumbar spine's posterior elements.

The question of whether or not these devices actually help has received an equivocal response. Although some back and neck pain sufferers have indicated that the devices did in fact help them, many physicians suggest that wearing these devices might, in the long run even worsen your condition. If you decide to pursue the use of one of these devices, we recommend that you proceed cautiously. You should wear one only after having undergone a thorough clinical examination by an experienced physician and a reasonable trial of less expensive therapy.

Traction

Traction involves some method for pulling the upper and lower parts of your body in opposite directions to ease your back or neck pain. The machinery used to perform the traction ranges from weights, harnesses and pulleys to canvas slings (gravity lumbar reduction devices). Proponents of traction claim that it is an effective therapy because it allows you to "stretch" the various elements of the spine, thereby reducing the pressure on the affected nerves. Furthermore, they suggest that traction force can also be directed in a manner that helps to realign the joints of your back into their proper positions. This latter perceived characteristic is closely akin to what is supposed to occur with spinal manipulation. The protocol for applying traction varies from continuously for several hours to intermittent bouts for seconds or minutes. The amount of resistance (pull) typically used for traction for lower back pain ranges from 15 to as much as several hundred pounds. Cervical traction for neck pain usually is 5-15 pounds. In the case of gravity lumbar reduction devices, your body's own weight is designed to do the work of the external force.

Considerable debate exists regarding whether or not traction is a useful form of therapy for back pain. Some physicians support its use, whereas others are adamantly against it. Whether to use traction or not is a decision that you should make carefully. Keep in mind that whatever the benefits of traction, they are short-lived. Once you stop being pulled, tugged and stretched, the elements of your spine will most likely go back to their old positions. One final note: We recommend that you religiously avoid all forms of inverted traction (e.g., inversion boots). No particular benefit exists because of your inverted position. On the contrary, an inverted position may cause microscopic bleeding in your eyes or brain.

Exercise

Exercises for back and neck pain are designed to stretch and strengthen the muscles that support your spine, and to maintain flexibility in those muscles and other supporting structures. If you strengthen certain muscles and stretch certain ligaments, you will be better able to position your back so that the forces affecting your spine are better distributed, the pressure on your facet joints is reduced and the backward bulging of your discs is minimized. Remember that the strength of your spine can be attributed not to its bones, but to its musculature and the binding (harnessing) effects of its ligaments and connective tissues.

There is seemingly wide consensus on the value of exercise to both treat and prevent back pain. Obviously, the primary focus of exercising involves the prevention of back pain.

The use of exercises as a means for preventing back pain is discussed at length in Chapter 6. Chapter 6 also includes a review of the traditional exercises used to develop the musculature supporting both your back (stretching exercises, abdominal exercises and lower back exercises) and your neck. Procedures for organizing an exercise program to prevent back and neck pain are also presented in Chapter 6.

Physical Therapy

Physical therapists are individuals trained in the treatment and prevention of musculoskeletal injuries, including back and neck pain. They are located at hospitals, clinics and private offices. They utilize many of the therapies and modalities mentioned on the previous pages, including heat/cold, diathermy, ultrasound, electrical stimulation, massage and traction. They can also show you exercises to do for your back and neck and how to correctly do them. Most states require a doctor's prescription for a physical therapist to treat you. If you have a serious enough problem with your back or neck, your injury is not improving with time, or you have a condition that might benefit from physical therapy, your doctor might recommend physical therapy for you.

Invasive Methods

Invasive methods for treating back pain involve techniques in which your body is invaded (entered) in some way. Acupuncture, trigger point injections, cortisone and Novocain injections and chemonucleolysis are the most common types of invasive methods. Although each of the techniques described in this section have brought relief to some individuals, we recommend that you remember that every invasive medical procedure carries some degree of medical risk.

Acupuncture. Acupuncture has evolved out of three thousand years of Chinese culture and history, and it entails placing thin needles at specific points of your body in order to dull or mask you back pain. The placement of the needles is arranged along lines of energy, called meridians, that run up, down and around your body, and have purportedly been mapped out over thousands of years by Chinese doctors. In some instances, the needles are supplemented by a low-voltage electrical current. Acupuncture has produced equivocal results. Some individuals swear by its effectiveness, while others claim not to have been helped by the procedure. In support of the former conclusion, some studies have indicated that acupuncture stimulates your body's production of endorphins, thereby relieving your back or neck pain.

Trigger Point Injections. Trigger point treatment involves injecting a local anesthetic into specific points that have been identified as producing pain in your back or neck. Numbing the trigger points (unduly sensitive areas) in your back or neck by means of injections is believed to somehow break up the pain cycle. A considerable degree of uncertainty surrounds this method of back treatment. Like acupuncture, the results are mixed—it works well for some, and not at all for others. In addition, in some instances, a simple saline solution or simply needling the trigger point without injecting anything at all has been found to be as successful in treating pain as an actual injection.

Cortisone Injections. Cortisone is a type of steroid medicine that works as a strong anti-inflammatory agent. Cortisone is injected in hopes of halting local inflammation. Cortisone can be used for trigger point injections, deep injections or for epidural injections. If your pain is well localized (such as a trigger point) and is due to inflammation, a cortisone shot can give significant relief to your pain.

Epidural cortisone injections consist of injecting cortisone into the spinal canal in the area surrounding the spinal cord and nerves (the epidural space). This procedure is similar to a spinal anesthetic. If the pain in your back and the pain going down into your leg are the result of localized inflammation in the epidural space and of the spinal nerves, an epidural cortisone shot can give dramatic relief. This is especially true when there is a bulging disc or degenerative arthritis causing spinal stenosis. Epidural cortisone injections usually are not of much help with a herniated disc.

Chemonucleolysis. Chemonucleolysis is a nonsurgical method for treating herniated or bulging discs. It involves injecting an enzyme, chymopapain, into the center portion of an injured disc. The enzyme, once injected, dissolves the nucleus (disc center) only, without affecting the adjacent outer portion of the disc, the nerves, the muscles and the ligaments. Dissolving the nucleus has been found to reduce the pressure (and thereby the pain) on the nerves near the disc. It should work better for a bulging disc than a herniated disc, where fragments of the disc may be within the spinal canal. The entire procedure for performing chemonucleolysis (from start to finish) takes about an hour and may require hospitalization afterwards. This therapy is certainly not risk-free, as very serious allergic reactions to the enzyme have occurred. Its success rate is comparable to other nonsurgical techniques. Chemonucleolysis has fallen into disfavor in recent years and is no longer commonly used.

Psychological Treatments

Few people realize just how closely their bodies and minds are intertwined. Each of us is, after all, just one organism. Studies have shown that specific psychologically focused therapies can be effective in treating back pain in certain instances. In general, these therapies fall into two groups. The first category involves efforts to relieve tension. If you relieve tension, you decrease the amount of muscular activity. When your muscle is tense, it is contracted. This contraction affects your nerves as well. Tension involves contraction, which in turn results in fatigue and pain because your nerves become electrically irritated. Eventually, you may experience excessive nervous tension, as well as excessive muscular tension. Too much tension can lead to back pain. Controlling your level of tension is essentially a function of learning to relax. It should be noted that relaxation is the opposite of movement. Relaxation is reflected by a reduction or a complete absence of muscular activity in your voluntary muscles. A number of effective techniques for learning how to relax have been developed, including progressive relaxation, mind-to-muscle relaxation, meditation, autogenic training, breathing training and visualization.

The second group of psychologically focused therapies involves techniques designed to enable you to "control" and "manage" your pain. Somewhat similar to the aforementioned relaxation techniques, these methods also focus on reducing the amount of tension you have. In addition, they attempt to change the way you perceive pain so that you are better prepared to deal with your pain, if necessary. Unfortunately, there are no guarantees that everyone will live a pain-free life. Those who have pain must learn to live with it. Learning how to gain control over your pain and your attendant emotions can be an invaluable action on your part. There are a number of diverse "control-and-manage" pain therapies, including biofeedback, hypnosis, progressive relaxation, visualization and behavioral analysis.

Back Pain Schools/Pain Clinics

A relatively recent development in the search to identify an effective means of treating back pain has been the establishment of organizations known generally as back pain schools or pain clinics. These organizations combine education with treatment within a setting of professional expertise and human understanding. Participation in the programs offered by these groups is designed to allow back pain sufferers to meet each other in a supportive and positive way. The treatment programs in these schools focus on educating you to accept responsibility for caring for your back, training you in the proper techniques for protecting your back and teaching you how to deal safely with the daily demands of your work and life. By offering the collective expertise of a diverse faculty of specialists and experts on back care, these clinics have been found to be a reasonable, effective, nonsurgical means of treating pain. In many instances they have proven to be more successful than other nonsurgical methods.

SURGICAL THERAPIES

Surgery serves a useful, but limited, function in treating back pain. In the vast majority of cases in which individuals suffer from back pain, surgery is not only unnecessary, but useless. There are only a few times when back surgery is essential. One is when pressure on a nerve must be diminished to relieve unmanageable pain. Another is when progressive nerve damage and paralysis must be halted. A third time is when there is painful motion in the spinal column that must be stopped to prevent recurrence of pain. There are also other, unusual circumstances in which your back pain may not be relieved within a reasonable period of time using nonsurgical therapies, and surgery is warranted. Whatever the problem is, though, it should have been present long enough to assume that nature alone is not going to treat it, and, in addition, nonsurgical therapies must have been tried and been unsuccessful. Finally, reasonable evidence should exist that surgery will correct, eliminate or improve your condition. Although no simple equation exists to give you an answer about whether or not your should have surgery, we strongly recommend that you adhere to the following advice: "If the risks involved in your surgery are high and the odds it will help are, at least in your opinion, low, it shouldn't be done."

The primary task of your physician, with regard to the question of whether or not you should have surgery, is to ensure that you are given sufficient information to make an informed decision. Cold statistics are one thing; your quality of life is quite another. The better informed you are, the more likely you will make a decision that is appropriate to your situation.

Once you and your physician have reached the decision that surgery is the best course of action for you, the type of surgery performed depends entirely on your condition. These procedures range from laminectomy (disc excision) to salvage back surgery (multiple back operations).

Laminectomy/Disc Removal

The most common surgical procedure for back pain is a laminectomy with disc removal. A laminectomy involves making a small opening in the lamina (the bone that is part of the vertebra which covers the affected level of the spinal canal). Once your physician can get at the slipped or herniated disc material that is pressing on the nerve root, it is removed. Any loose fragments within the space between the vertebrae or within the disc are also removed to prevent the possibility of the recurrence of pain. The operation, conducted with the patient under some type of anesthesia, normally takes anywhere from 30 to 90 minutes in the average-sized individual. Following surgery, you may be hospitalized for a short period of time. After your discharge from the hospital, you should be able to resume full-time work in approximately three to four weeks. Full recovery (the operation is fully forgotten) usually takes about six months. The success rate for this type of surgical therapy is often as high as 90 percent.

Spinal Fusion

Spinal fusion, a special type of back surgery, is an operation in which bone from somewhere else in your body, or from a donor's body, is grafted onto living bone in your back. Eventually the grafted bone in your body will be replaced by living bone produced by your body. In the meantime, you have made a strong, stable union between two or more vertebrae (the bones selected for fusion). This stable union eliminates motion at that particular segment of your spine. Any pain that had previously been produced or irritated by the excessive or abnormal motion that existed will subside. The success rate of spinal fusion operations has not been found to be above the host of nonsurgical therapies discussed previously. For that reason, the incidence of spinal fusions has decreased dramatically in recent years. Except in instances in which the likely benefits of a spinal fusion are well-documented (e.g., following a severe spinal fracture in which the joints between the vertebrae are so severely injured that the stability of your spine is in question), the possible negative complications from a spinal fusion should be weighed against the potential benefits.

Surgery To Relieve Spinal Stenosis

Spinal stenosis is a condition in which the space in your spinal canal is not big enough. This condition can be congenital. More often, though, it is the result of arthritis and bone spurs in your vertebral bodies or facet joints that cause narrowing of the spinal canal. Stenosis can also be caused by a degenerative or a herniated disc. The surgical procedure for this condition involves removing any and all structures that are impinging on the nerves within the spinal canal. If the need for this operation is confirmed beforehand by radiographic studies (myelogram, MRI, or a CAT scan), the operation is usually successful. Spinal stenosis occurs more often in older individuals.

Surgery To Treat Infections

Infections of the spine can be quite painful. Although antibiotics alone can often eliminate such infections, in some instances surgery may be necessary to treat them. In these cases, surgery is performed to drain the infection and to remove enough of the soft tissue and bone to cure the infection while maintaining as much of the spine as possible. A thorough cleansing of the area with a sterile solution containing antibiotics is also done to prevent recurrence of the infection. In some cases, depending upon how much of the bone had to be removed, a bone graft may subsequently be required to fuse and reconstruct the spine.

Surgery To Remove Tumors

The decision on whether or not to surgically remove a tumor must be made taking several factors into account. Can it be treated with chemotherapy or radiation? Is it benign or malignant? Did it originate in your spine, or has it migrated from elsewhere in your body? What are the risks involved in surgery for this specific tumor? What are the probable outcomes of both performing and not performing this surgery? In general, the procedures of this type of surgery are similar to those for surgery to treat infections. Because the surgeon has to eliminate all of the tumor plus an appropriate margin of normal spine adjacent to the tumor, the surgical risks and skills needed to perform the operation successfully are substantially higher when operating to remove a tumor than for treating a spinal infection. The likelihood of needing a bone graft or other type of spinal replacement device or material to rebuild the spine after this operation is also increased.

Surgery To Treat Injuries

Many fractures of your spine will heal with good function and without long-lasting significant pain, just as fractures heal elsewhere in your body. Whether or not surgery is required depends on the extent of bony and ligamentous damage. An important factor in the decision-making process for surgically treating spine fractures is whether the fracture is stable or unstable. If the fracture is stable (e.g. a compression fracture in the thoracic spine), it should heal without surgery. If the fracture is unstable, injury to the spinal cord and nerves can or has occurred. Unstable fractures are treated surgically to stabilize the injured area of spine and to prevent or correct injury to the spinal cord and nerves. Even in someone with an unstable fracture and paralysis, surgery is usually performed to stabilize the injured area, prevent further damage and allow the patient to start sitting or getting up. If surgery is required, the operation performed is a spinal fusion with the placement of stainless steel rods or plates that span the injured area. The rods or plates are held by screws or hooks that are placed into the bones of the spine.

Salvage Back Surgery

Salvage back surgery is surgery that is performed on someone who has already had two or more operations for back pain. Numerous studies suggest that additional surgical operations often have decreasing chances of success. As a result, except in those extremely rare circumstances when multiple back operations are warranted, you should be very cautious before undergoing surgery again.

THE NEXT STEP

The first four chapters of this book examined the basics of back pain: an anatomical overview of your back; the causes of back pain; how your doctor diagnoses and evaluates your back pain; and the most common nonsurgical and surgical therapies for treating back pain. Chapter 5 presents a discussion of how the Tempur-Pedic mattress and neck pillow can help you get a good night's sleep.

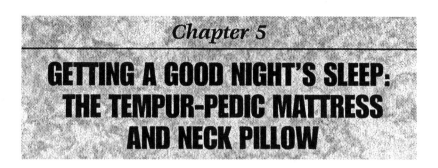

GETTING A GOOD NIGHT'S SLEEP: THE TEMPUR-PEDIC MATTRESS AND NECK PILLOW

"It's a funny thing about life; if you refuse to accept anything but the best, you often get it."
—Somerset Maugham

O ne thing that is routinely overlooked by most people as a contributing factor to our health is the bed that we sleep on. Statistics indicate that we spend about one third of our lives asleep in our bedroom. The quality of our sleep greatly affects the other two thirds of our life while we are awake. The notion that the sleeping surface we use can affect our well-being is somewhat foreign to most people. In fact, many people have grown accustomed to a less-than-comfortable bed on which they toss and turn all night and wake up stiff and sore.

Surprisingly, when you think about sleep, many people have willingly accepted something less than satisfactory in this high-tech society in which we live. About 90% of us sleep on inner spring mattresses, which were introduced in the 1920s as a breakthrough in mattress technology. Since then, almost every aspect of our lives has been touched by dramatic advancements in product technology (e.g., automobiles, airplanes, computer software and hardware, VCR's, etc.). These advancements have not occurred overnight. Rather, most product categories have gone through several major development periods. Audio products, for example, have evolved from vinyl records to 8-track tapes to cassettes to CD's.

A few products, however, have not participated in the technological revolution. Mattresses, for example, where we spend one third of our lives, have experienced little or no progression of improvement. We are basically sleeping on the same type of surface that our parents and our grandparents slept on in the 1920s. To be sure, some minor improvements to inner spring mattresses have been made in past years, but these (if anything) were essentially cosmetic in nature. Except for the introduction of a few limited market alternatives (e.g., waterbeds and air mattresses), no fundamental change or major leap forward in technology has occurred in the mattress industry.

Waterbeds were introduced and became quite popular in the 1970s as an alternative to traditional inner springs. Since—by definition—these mattresses are closed systems, they have specific limiting features, including the fact that they make many people perspire profusely. The same can be said about some air mattresses that have been introduced in recent years.

A significant advancement in hospital mattress technology, however, has taken place. Super expensive, low-air loss and air-fluidized beds (ranging in price from $2,000 to $200,000) were developed to combat pressure sores. Although these units are effective at providing pressure relief, they have several limiting features. For example, they are expensive to buy or rent, have high maintenance costs and require constant supervision. Accordingly, mattresses designed specifically for hospitals are impractical for use in the home by the general public.

TEMPUR-PEDIC: THE STORY

Before now, an affordable product has not been available to the general public which could provide the type of pressure relief provided by a hospital mattress. The Tempur-Pedic mattress—featuring Tempur Foam—has changed this situation. Tempur Foam is the result of 10 years of trial and error research conducted by Fagerdala World Foams of Varmdo, Sweden in their Danish manufacturing facility. The original "Temper" Foam was developed for NASA with the idea of producing a material which would cushion airplane pilots and astronauts during landings and take off. Unfortunately, the material that evolved from those efforts was very difficult to control in the manufacturing process and to make in different sizes and shapes. Although the potential benefits of this material were relatively well known at that time, most companies ceased production of the product because of the aforementioned issues.

A Swedish group, however, was intrigued by the inherent possibilities of such a foam product and spent millions of dollars attempting to improve the foam and mass produce it. The effort succeeded. The group began testing it in the late 1980s in Swedish and Danish hospitals. Medical researchers quickly found that, in addition to being very effective at treating and preventing pressure sores in these facilities, this product was uniquely well suited to patients that had back or joint pain. The product was launched to the Swedish public in the fall of 1991, and it proved to be an instant hit. This innovative product has tremendously impacted the mattress market in Sweden, witness the fact that over 30,000 mattresses have been sold per year in a country of only eight million people. In 1992, Tempur-Pedic, Inc. of Lexington, Kentucky was formed to import and distribute the products throughout the United States (Figure 1). In addition to Sweden and the United States, Tempur-Pedic products are now being sold in 15 other countries in both Europe and Asia.

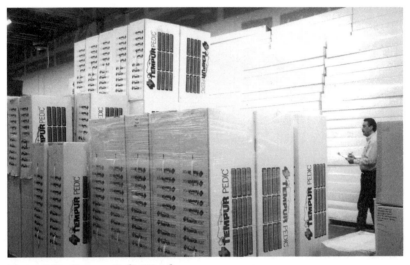

Figure 5-1   Tempur-Pedic Warehouse

THE TEMPUR-PEDIC MATTRESS: THE NEXT LEAP FORWARD

The Tempur-Pedic Swedish Mattress is the long overdue leap forward in technology that restless sleepers and back pain sufferers have needed and deserved. This product, since its introduction in Sweden to the general public in 1991, has been thoroughly tested in both Europe and the United States and has been found to be a unique pressure relieving sleep surface. The Tempur-Pedic material is a viscoelastic, temperature reactive, open-cell foam (Figure 5-2). Due to its open-cell structure and its ability to breathe, the Tempur-Pedic Mattress never feels warm and never causes users to perspire.

At first contact, the Tempur-Pedic Mattress feels quite firm. When it is exposed to the temperature and weight of a human body, however, it is readily compressed. When pressure is removed, the mattress slowly resumes its shape. In other words, the material actually conforms to the body instead of pressing against it like almost any other conventional surface (Figure 5-3). This molding effect distrib-

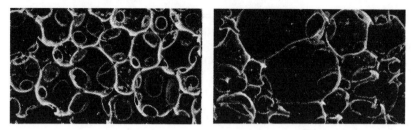

Figure 5-2   Left, Tempur-Pedic Foam; Right, Standard High Resilient Foam

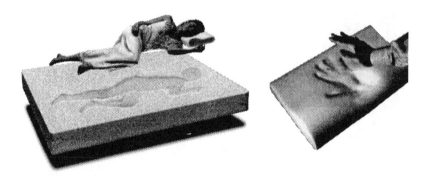

Figure 5-3   Sample of impression made on Tempur-Pedic with equal pressure on all points.

utes pressure evenly over the entire supported surface. The highly desirable end product of the pressure relief is the comfort the Tempur-Pedic Mattress provides.

With conventional bedding, points exist on the body that have more pressure than others; hence the term "pressure points" (Figure 5-4). The primary reason an individual tosses and turns at night is a slow down of the blood supply to certain areas (pressure points) of the body that are in contact with the mattress. The brain recognizes this and instructs the body to move in order to maintain capillary (tiny blood vessels) blood flow. With the even distribution of pressure provided by the Tempur-Pedic Mattress, capillary blood supply to those parts of the body in contact with the mattress is maintained at a much higher level. The end result is less tossing and turning and a much more restful night's sleep.

Numerous clinical and scientific studies have documented the effectiveness of the Tempur-Pedic Mattress. At the Institute for Clinical and Physiologic Research at Lillhagan Hospital in Gothenburg, Sweden, it was conclusively demonstrated that patients tossed and turned an average of 17 times per night on the Tempur-Pedic Mattress versus 80-100 times on a standard mattress. At the Twin City Testing Corporation in St. Paul, Minnesota, research on body interface pressure points was performed on the Tempur-Pedic Mattress. In this study, pressures on certain parts of the body were noted to be well below the medically

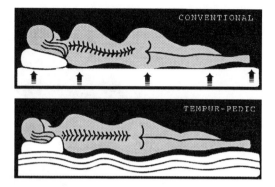

A conventional mattress (top) forces your body into an unnatural position, while Tempur-Pedic (bottom) keeps your spine in perfect alignment.

Figure 5-4   Pressure Points

and industry accepted standards for pressure reduction and pressure relief for support surfaces (mattresses). Computer testing, using electronic devices to measure the pressure distribution of a human body lying on a bed, has been conducted to compare the Tempur-Pedic Swedish Mattress with a top-of-the-line spring mattress. The results of this testing show that the best pressure relief (by far) was obtained with the Tempur-Pedic Mattress—a result that was true for people of either gender (Figure 5-5). Furthermore, an investigation at the University of Maine showed that children aged 5-10 had significantly greater levels of deep sleep while sleeping on a Tempur-Pedic Mattress as compared to a standard mattress.

Although the Tempur-Pedic Mattress was initially designed for people with back and joint pain, sleep problems and pressure sores, the mattress is also well suited to anyone who wants a more restful night's sleep. Furthermore, people with minor aches and pains associated with chronic conditions or sports injuries reported a significant decrease in morning stiffness. They also seem to sleep better and toss and turn less. These anecdotal studies, as well as the clinical and scientific studies performed, lend further credence to the manufacturer's claims.

After working with the product for several years, the authors have come to view the Tempur-Pedic Swedish Mattress as an extraordinary improvement to traditional sleep surfaces from an orthopedic viewpoint. It is helpful in the prevention of back problems because it supports and places the spine in correct alignment while sleeping. It is also helpful in minimizing pain associated with chronic joint or

Pressure analysis on innerspring mattress indicates higher pressure and less comfort. (higher peaks represent higher pressure).

INNER-SPRING

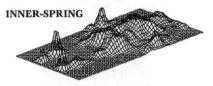

Pressure analysis on Tempur-Pedic shows even distribution of body weight for perfect support!

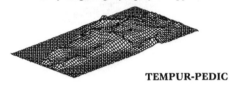

TEMPUR-PEDIC

Figure 5-5   Raised Area Grid

back conditions. Finally, it facilitates healing of the nagging injuries that many of us have to live with from time to time. In other words, the Tempur-Pedic Mattress is a remarkable product that offers substantial benefits to a wide array of users.

THE TEMPUR-PEDIC NECK PILLOW

The Tempur-Pedic Mattress is best used in conjunction with the Tempur-Pedic Swedish Neck Pillow made from the same material. This pillow has proven to be an exceptionally popular product in the United States particularly for individuals with neck problems. For these individuals, the important factor in achieving pain relief is to reinforce the neck area during periods of rest by building up support to the natural curve of the upper spine.

The benefits of using a Tempur-Pedic Neck Pillow are substantial. For example, the anatomically correct shape and unique pain relieving properties of the Tempur-Pedic Neck Pillow enable individuals with neck and back discomfort to get a better night's sleep (Figure 5-6). Placing the head, neck and spine in correct cervical alignment and eliminating high pressure contact points provide maximum pressure relief and support, allowing the neck, shoulder and upper back muscles to relax completely. For individuals with back, neck, shoulder or other joint pain, using the Tempur-Pedic Swedish Mattress and the Tempur-Pedic Neck Pillow should be one of the first steps in their comprehensive treatment program.

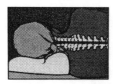

TEMPUR-PEDIC NECK PILLOW

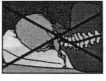

ORDINARY PILLOW

Figure 5-6   Tempur-Pedic Neck Pillow

OTHER TEMPUR-PEDIC PRODUCTS

The Tempur-Pedic Lumbar Pad is a lower back support pad which should be used by individuals who must sit for a prolonged period of time or by those who have low back pain when sitting for even short periods of time. It has proven effective in treating and preventing lower back pain in a wide variety of individuals who must sit while they work, for example, secretaries, long distance truck drivers, bus drivers, airplane pilots, etc. The scientifically unique foam in the Tempur-Pedic Lumbar Pad gently molds to the shape of your lower back, thereby relieving pressure on your back as it helps retain the natural curve of your spine.

The Tempur-Pedic Comfort Cushion is another unequalled product from Tempur-Pedic, Inc. This cushion can be used on any sitting surface to make that surface feel custom built for comfort. The Tempur-Pedic Comfort Cushion molds to the shape of your buttocks, not only to provide support, but also to enable your weight to be evenly distributed while you're sitting. Collectively, the net effect of using the Tempur-Pedic Comfort Cushion is the prevention or relief of low back, tail bone, buttock or sciatic-type pain caused by sitting.

The medical division of Tempur-Pedic, Inc. also distributes directly to hospitals and nursing homes throughout the USA. The Tempur-Med Hospital Mattress is rapidly becoming the mattress of choice for those hospitals which have made a serious commitment about treating and preventing pressure sores. Not surprisingly, the

Tempur-Med Mattress is a very attractive alternative to the previously mentioned low air-loss and air-fluidized beds. The Tempur-Med Wheel-chair Cushion is also rapidly gaining respect in the market place as the best and most cost efficient pressure relieving wheelchair cush-ion available.

Today, the Tempur-Pedic Mattress, the Tempur-Pedic Neck Pil-low, and other products are sold through a network of over 5,000 doc-tors of chiropractic, medical doctors and physical therapists through-out the United States and more than 15,000 medical professionals worldwide. These products are also sold directly to the public by Tempur-Pedic, Inc. and through specialty bed and back stores nation-ally. For additional information on any Tempur-Pedic product, you can call 1-800-886-6466 or write:

Tempur-Pedic, Inc.
848 G Nandino Blvd.
Lexington, KY 40511

BROOKSTONE

The largest retailer of the Tempur-Pedic products is Brookstone which has more than 140 outlets in major malls in highly populated cities. The best way to see the product firsthand is to visit one of the Brookstone stores where a Tempur-Pedic Mattress and Tempur-Pedic Neck Pillow are displayed—complete with product brochures and vid-eos.

For more information on the Brookstone store nearest you call: Brookstone customer service at 1-800-846-3000.

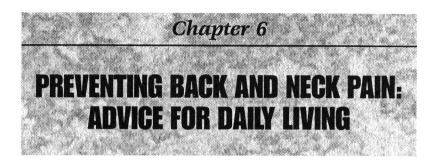

Chapter 6

PREVENTING BACK AND NECK PAIN: ADVICE FOR DAILY LIVING

"To take what there is, and use it, without waiting forever in vain
for the preconceived—to dig deep into the actual and get some-
thing out of that—this doubtless is the right way to live."
—Henry James

This chapter is for people at various stages of back or neck pain or recovery from it. It presents basic guidelines on how to take care of your back or neck properly after you've recovered from a bout of pain and want to avoid a recurrence. It is also for you to consult when your pain is in the process of subsiding and you want to do whatever is feasible to expedite the process. Finally, it offers general suggestions to individuals who have never had back or neck pain on what to do to maximize their chances of avoiding it.

As you can readily see, almost everyone can identify with one of the three aforementioned categories. Either you've had back or neck pain in the past and would like to avoid another bout in the future, you currently have back or neck pain and want to get rid of it as painlessly and as quickly as possible, or you've never had back or neck pain and want to continue in that fortunate state for the foreseeable future. Our advice to each person is the same: "Identify an appropriate plan for your daily living to enable you to achieve your goal and follow your plan." In other words, develop a strategic plan for your life. The critical elements of such a plan are the same for all three categories of individuals. First, learn what makes good sense concerning your spine as you perform all your customary daily tasks. Second, reduce the load that your spine must carry around and your muscles must support by shedding excess poundage. Third, engage in a properly designed exercise program to stretch and strengthen your back or neck muscles and the muscles supporting your spine. Fourth, if you are a woman, be aware of the fact that there are some spine-related problems that only women have. You should design your "strategic" plan for daily living accordingly.

GOOD SENSE REGARDING CUSTOMARY TASKS

If you are serious about avoiding back and neck pain, you must take some care in how you go about performing your "normal" tasks. Biomechanically, there is a proper way that these activities should be performed if you wish to keep the stresses on your spine and your back and neck muscles to a minimum. Increasing the stresses can result in a corresponding increase in the likelihood that you will encounter back or neck pain at some point in your life. Accordingly, you should adhere as closely as possible to steps that will minimize stress on your spine, whatever the task.

Posture

Your first step in preventing back and neck pain is to maintain good posture in all of your body's positions. Failure to do so will place undesirable stress on your spine. Understanding a simple law of physics can explain why this is so. This law states that when a force is applied to a curved structure, the greatest stress is applied on the inner (concave) side of the curve. As a result, the greater the curve in your spine, the more uneven the amount of pressure over your spine, with the largest force concentrated at the apex of the curve. In turn, this circumstance then results in excessive wear on your intervertebral joints at the apex of the curve of your spine. This excessive wear may subsequently cause your lower back (for example) to be affected earlier than normal by degenerative changes or wear-and-tear factors.

It is not difficult to comprehend why individuals with good posture are less likely to suffer back and neck pain or be injured than individuals with poor posture. Individuals with poor posture put too much strain on their backs and necks by localizing too much of the stress on one area of their spine. Individuals with good posture are able to distribute more of the forces being applied to their spine throughout their entire spine.

Good posture is essential whether you're standing, sitting, bending over, rising up, sleeping or performing any of your many daily activities. Fortunately, as we saw countless times among the cadets at the United States Military Academy while we were on the USMA faculty, good posture is not very difficult to achieve.

Standing. Good posture (while standing) involves holding your head high while simultaneously tucking in your chin. This action flattens the curve in your cervical spine. You should also pull your stomach in, roll your hips slightly backward (thereby tilting your pelvis slightly backward) and tighten your buttock muscles somewhat

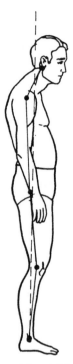

- Hold your head high. Tuck your chin in slightly. Stand tall.
- Relax your shoulders. Elevate your chest slightly. Hold your abdomen in. Your beltline should be horizontal to the ground.
- Bring your hips back over your ankles. Tuck your pelvis (tailbone) down.
- Keep your knees straight but not locked.
- Rock forward and back. Place your weight on your feet in the area in front of your ankle bone.

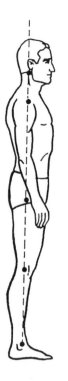

Figure 6-1   Achieving good posture

by contracting (squeezing) them (Figure 6-1). This maneuver flattens the curve in your lumbar spine. Remember that good posture begins with your head and your pelvis—get them properly aligned and the rest of your body will fall into line. If you must stand for an extended period of time, don't stand in the same position for too long. You should periodically shift your weight and change positions. You should also support one foot above the other on a low stool or box, alternating your feet every so often.

Sitting. A proper sitting position is important—both at work and during periods of relaxation. The best basic position is one in which you keep your knees level with your hips and your feet flat on the floor. Your back should be firmly supported by the back of your chair. This support enables you to maintain the lordotic curve in your lower back without undue muscular effort on your part. The support can be provided by an external device (e.g., a Tempur-Pedic Lumbar Pad, a small pillow or a rolled-up towel) or by an orthopedically designed chair (e.g., one with lumbar back support built into it). If possible, the chair in which you choose to sit should have armrests, because the support provided by armrests helps to ease the load on your spine. Your chair should be adjustable in height so that you can attain the proper sitting position (especially if you have a job in which you sit most of the day). You should get up from your chair for five minutes at least once every half hour and move around. You should avoid slouching down in your chair. Although a slouched position may seem comfortable, it actually places additional stress on your back and neck. You should sit back in your chair with your head held directly over your shoulders. As much as possible, you should also avoid leaning forward while sitting to work at a desk or table.

Sleeping. Since most of us spend approximately one-third of our lives in bed, it is little wonder that much has been written about choosing a mattress. To make the decision "easier" for you, manufacturers of mattresses frequently attach adjectives such as "orthopedic," "chiropractic" and "posture" to their products. The inference is obvious. Reportedly, these products—described in "medical" terms—have been scientifically designed and tested for anyone who cares to provide the best care for their spine. The truth of the situation is often another matter.

In the first place, in general, no hard-and-fast rules exist with regard to the selection of a mattress. As simple as it sounds, what is best is whatever works best for you. Since most individuals suffering from back pain find a soft (sagging) bed to be uncomfortable, the traditional rule of thumb is that a relatively firm mattress is recommended for back pain sufferers. Some people, however, prefer a mattress that is less firm or even soft. You should test a variety of mattresses until you find one that is comfortable for your spine. (Refer to Chapter 5 for a comprehensive discussion of how the features of a Tempur-Pedic Mattress can help an individual prevent and treat back pain).

In addition to selecting a mattress that is appropriate to your needs, you also should find a comfortable sleeping position. If you try a position and it isn't comfortable, try another. As a general rule, if you suffer from back or neck pain, you should avoid sleeping on your stomach, since this position tends to exaggerate both the curve in your lower back and the curve in your cervical spine, thereby placing an unnecessary strain on your spine. If you tend to sleep on your back, we recommend that you place a pillow under your knees and a pillow under your neck. If you sleep on your side, you should bend your knees. If you are currently suffering from either back or neck pain, you should use as many pillows as necessary to keep your spine level while you sleep. A sagging spine can exacerbate the pain in your back or neck. Your shoulders and hips should be in a vertical line.

If you're in pain, you should also decide what is the best way to get into and out of bed. The general rule of thumb is to do both movements slowly and gradually. Pain has a very sharp way of letting you know if you move too suddenly or too unknowingly. To get into bed, first sit on the side of the bed with your palms resting on the mattress. Then slowly lower your body sideways and simultaneously raise your legs so you end up lying on your side. Use your hands and then your forearms to ease your movements from sitting to lying, making every effort to avoid putting stress on your spine. Once you are on your side, slowly move into your favorite position for sleeping. Getting out of bed simply involves doing the movements for getting into bed in reverse order. You should avoid twisting or bending your back while getting into or out of bed.

Walking. Good posture while walking involves the same basic elements of correct posture that standing does. Stand tall. Hold your head high and neck directly over your shoulders. Keep your chin tucked in slightly. Pull your stomach in. Roll your hips slightly backward. Tighten your buttock muscles. If you carry a shoulder bag as you walk, switch the bag from shoulder to shoulder periodically.

Lifting. Many back injuries are caused by improper lifting techniques. As a general rule, you can avoid these injuries by being aware of and adhering to the 12 basic rules of lifting.

1. Stand close to the object you're lifting with your feet apart to ensure that you have firm footing.
2. Bend your knees. Keep your back as straight as possible by minimizing any bending at your waist. Bending at the waist increases the stress on your back.
3. Tighten your stomach muscles before you lift. Your abdominal muscles, as we mentioned in Chapter 1, can be considered as your anterior back muscles. They help to support your back.
4. Lift with your legs by slowly straightening them. Make your legs (not your back muscles) do the work.
5. Hold the (lifted) load close to your body. The farther away an object is held from your body, the greater the stress it will place on your back.
6. Keep your back in an upright position and avoid leaning your head forward during the lift and while holding the object.
7. Reverse steps #1 through #6 to lower your load.
8. Avoid twisting your body while lifting. Move your feet if it's necessary to change directions or to see something not otherwise in view.
9. While carrying an object, move smoothly. Don't move suddenly or jerk your body.
10. Decide where you're going to go with the object you're going to lift before you lift it. Make sure that you have a clear path to reach that point before you lift the object.
11. Check the object to be lifted carefully for any possible impediments (e.g., a sharp or jagged edge) before you lift the object.
12. Get assistance if the object to be lifted is too heavy or large.

Traveling. Guidelines for maintaining proper body mechanics while traveling depend on your mode of travel. If you're driving a car, we recommend that you push your car seat into a comfortable position as far forward as possible, so you can avoid over-reaching for the pedals. Whether you're the driver or a passenger in a car, you might consider putting a Tempur-Pedic Lumbar Pad or a rolled-up towel behind your lower back to support it. If your car seats are very soft and you prefer a more rigid seat, you should consider purchasing some type of device that will provide that rigidity (e.g. a Tempur-Pedic Comfort Cushion). These devices vary widely in both cost and complexity. If you have to be in the car for an extended period of time, you should stop every hour or so and get out to stretch and walk around.

If you're traveling by plane, there are several options to consider in order to maintain a good position for your spine. Like auto travel, you can place one or more small pillows (readily available on most commercial flights) behind your lower back and neck to provide support. If you are short, you may find it necessary to take a carry-on piece of luggage to be used to prop up your feet once the flight is airborne. If you are tall, you should make every effort to get an aisle seat so that you can stretch your legs occasionally. You should also ask the reservations/seat assignment person if it would be possible to assign you a seat with extra leg room. On commercial flights, such seats are often adjacent to emergency exits and are called bulkhead seats. But whatever your height, you should periodically get up and walk around during the flight.

Sports

In the environment in which we previously worked at West Point, almost everyone—cadets, staff and faculty and dependents—was an athlete of some sort. Ranging from the intercollegiate competitive sports teams for the cadets to the recreational noontime joggers, the vast majority of the West Point community engages in some level of regular physical activity. While the degree of enthusiasm for athletics or personal conditioning may not be quite as extensive or intense in your community, it would not be surprising if the majority of people you know like to work out or participate in some form of physical activity.

Individuals who fall into the aforementioned category face several basic questions regarding the possible effects that physical exertion has on the health of their spine. What is the possible danger to your spine from participating in a specific sport or conditioning activity? Is there anything that you can or should do to protect your spine while participating? Is there anything that you can do before participating that will subsequently help your spine?

Listing all the possible sports and conditioning activities in which you could engage would be a substantial undertaking. Developing a checklist of possible beneficial guidelines to protect your back and neck while participating in those activities would be an even more extensive task. Identifying what you can do before you become an active participant is somewhat easier. Unquestionably, the most valuable action you can take is to get into as good a condition as possible. With regard to your spine, this task involves strengthening your abdominal, lower back, and neck muscles using a variety of the numerous exercises that can accomplish such an objective. Healthy muscles are not only strong, but flexible. Maintaining your flexibility should also be an important aspect of your conditioning program. (Note: Your choice of strengthening exercises for the spine is somewhat extensive. For example, there are over 30 separate calisthenic-type exercises for strengthening just the stomach muscles. The sit-up is probably the most common one, but there are others that are even more effective).

We also highly recommend that both before and while you are participating in sports and conditioning activities, you exercise a lot of common sense regarding your spine. Be sure you have stretched and warmed up before exercising. Don't take any unreasonable chances. Table 6-1 illustrates the relative risks of incurring a back or neck injury from participating in selected sports and fitness activities.

The question arises: What is reasonable? Obviously, "reasonable" is a relative term. What may be reasonable to us may be unreasonable to you. It's *your* back and neck, *your* life and *your* decision. Above all, we suggest, however, that you "listen" to your body. If either your back or neck hurts, your body is sending you a message. Don't ignore it. You may need to make some changes in what you're doing. Probably the most sensible advice we could give you is that when deciding whether or not to participate in a specific activity, you should consider the pleasure-pain ratio—a subjectively quantitative measure first suggested by Dr. Augustus White in his best-selling book, *Your Aching Back*. White recommended that if the pleasure you derive from a sport exceeds the back pain you incur, then have at it. Within the limits of common sense, we agree.

Sexual Activity

In sexual relations, as in every other form of physical activity, the principles of sensible spine care hold true. You and your partner must be aware of and use proper body mechanics while making love so as not to irritate your spine. As you may well know, when your back or neck pain is severe enough, movements associated with usual

HIGH-RISK ACTIVITIES	FOOTBALL GYMNASTICS POWER LIFTING WRESTLING
MEDIUM- TO HIGH-RISK ACTIVITIES	HANDBALL HOCKEY LACROSSE RACQUETBALL SQUASH
MEDIUM-RISK ACTIVITIES	BASEBALL DANCE DIVING ROWING SOCCER TRACK & FIELD —THROWING EVENTS —RUNNING
LOW- TO MEDIUM-RISK ACTIVITIES	BASKETBALL BOXING DOWNHILL SKIING GOLF JOGGING STRENGTH TRAINING TENNIS VOLLEYBALL
LOW-RISK ACTIVITIES	CROSS COUNTRY SKIING CYCLING SAILING SCUBA DIVING SWIMMING WALKING

Table 6-1   The relative risks of incurring a back injury from participating in selected sports and fitness activities*

*Note: You should keep in mind that there is a difference between relatively minor back pain that is muscle-related and a back injury. Participation in many of these sports and fitness activities can result in back pain; most, however, are not high risk in terms of their potential for causing back injury.

sexual activity may become almost impossible. Even when your back or neck pain is not that severe, your fear that sexual activity may make your pain worse can inhibit you emotionally. For the record, there is no cause or factor related to back or neck pain that is adversely affected by sexual activity. You need not fear that sex may, somehow, inflict permanent damage to your spine.

Having learned that your risk of physiological harm from sexual activity is very unlikely, you should also be aware that, for some people, back or neck pain has been known to cause either sexual dysfunction or make a preexisting sexual problem worse. There are isolated cases in which men have become impotent and women frigid because of back or neck pain. There are also instances in which back or neck pain has aggravated a preexisting state of emotional strain and hostility between individuals. In such cases, a loss of sex drive may result. In all of these examples, the problems are essentially psychologically (e.g., emotionally) rooted.

What you and your partner need in these instances is a proper mixture of clear, honest communication; trust; patience and sympathetic understanding. Individuals who haven't been able to achieve that mix (for whatever reason) are advised to seek professional assistance.

There are several guidelines that you should consider if you or your partner has a back or neck pain problem and you want to maintain a mutually satisfying sex life. For discussion purposes, these guidelines are grouped into two categories: consciousness and mechanical.

Consciousness Guidelines

1. Start with a positive attitude. Your back or neck pain is not going to keep you and your partner from having a satisfying sex life.
2. Talk to your partner. There simply is no substitute for honest, caring communication. Be as subtle or as frank as you'd like, but open the lines of direct communication as soon as possible.
3. Approach the problem of how to deal with back or neck pain (while maintaining a satisfying sex life) with a cooperative attitude. You and your partner must make a firm commitment to give and take, when necessary, to achieve the most satisfying experience for both of you. This approach will require a maximum degree of sympathetic understanding of what is pleasurable and what is painful for the other partner.
4. Be more open-minded about lovemaking. Expand your attitudes. Talk more. Touch more. Care more. Be more sensual. Lovemaking can, and should, involve more than coital activities.

5. Enjoy what you're doing while lovemaking if it doesn't hurt. If it does hurt, make a commitment to knowing and adhering to the following mechanical guidelines for making love when you have a back or neck problem.

Mechanical Guidelines

1. Don't bend forward at the waist with your knees straight during sexual intercourse. Even if you're lying down, this position puts tremendous stress on your lower back. If you bend your knees, you can bend slightly forward.
2. Arch your lower back as little as possible, because arching your back places considerable force on the posterior structures of your spine.
3. Don't lie flat on your stomach or your back with your hips extended straight. This position over-stresses the hip flexor muscles that extend from the front of your lumbar spine to just below your hip joint. If these muscles are tense or taut, pressure is put on your lower back. You can relax these muscles by bending at the hips; flex (bend) one or both of your hips. Assuming a hips-flexed position will help protect your lower back from irritation.
4. Don't bend your neck too far backwards or forward. Overly bending your neck (particularly backwards) may place excessive stress on the cervical curve of your spine.
5. Consider using one of the positions for sexual intercourse shown in Figures 6-5 to 6-9. Each of these positions is particularly suited for partners, one of whom has back or neck pain.

Once you understand and make a reasonable attempt to adhere to the aforementioned guidelines, is there anything else you can do? Keeping in mind that this text is not intended to be a lovemaking manual and that we are not particularly qualified to write one, we offer the following additional suggestions for you to consider. If you have back pain, your partner should be the one to provide any motion during sexual intercourse. If your pain is greater than your pleasure during lovemaking, then you or your partner must make an appropriate adaptation in either body position or technique. When you irritate your spine, pain is your body's way of keeping you informed that you're doing something that is over-stressing your back or neck. And finally, in view of the wide array of pleasurable alternatives for achieving a satisfying sex life, even for those individuals with back or neck pain, the old adage "where there's a will there's a way" may apply.

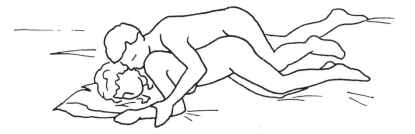

Figure 6-2   This is the traditional basic position when either partner suffers from back pain. It is possibly the best lovemaking position to use when either partner's back pain is in the acute stage.

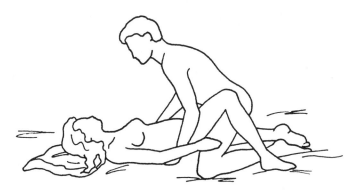

Figure 6-3   This position is good when the woman suffers from back pain. The woman's upper torso should be supported with pillows and her thighs should be supported by her partner's arms and thighs.

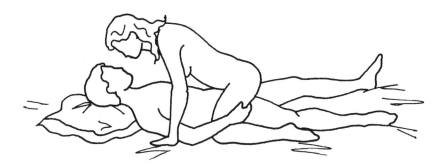

Figure 6-4   This position is good when the woman suffers back pain. This can also be a good position for a man with back pain, provided his upper torso is raised slightly (with pillows) in order to flex his spine.

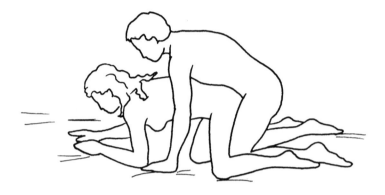

Figure 6-5   This position is good when the man suffers from back pain. Note that his back is slightly flexed, as opposed to extended. This is not a good position for a woman with back pain.

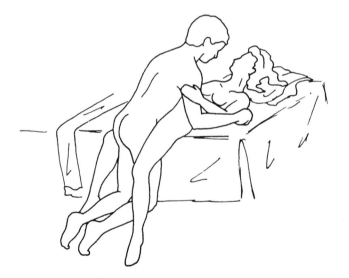

Figure 6-6   This position is good when the man suffers from back pain. This is not a good position when the woman has back pain.

MAINTAINING BODY LEANNESS

If by shedding extra pounds you reduce the load that your spine must carry around and your back muscles must support, you reduce the stress your back must handle. At the same time, you decrease the likelihood that you will suffer from back pain. Keeping your weight at an appropriate level can also have a positive effect on your posture. A protruding stomach frequently leads to lordosis (swayback), a condition that places considerable stress on the posterior elements of the spine. A flat, muscularly fit stomach, on the other hand, lends itself to the maintenance of proper body mechanics. As we mentioned earlier, your stomach muscles play an important role in supporting your back. For that reason, they are frequently referred to as your "anterior back muscles."

Before offering suggestions on how you might approach the process of shedding excess poundage, we'd like to explain the difference between two very important terms: overweight and overfat. It is important that you understand the precise meanings of these terms if you are to maintain body leanness. Being overweight simply means weighing more than other individuals of the same height and age. Being overfat, on the other hand, means you have more body fat than you should for your good health. Overfat is an indication of poor fitness. Overweight, on the other hand, is not an accurate indicator of fitness because some people simply have more muscle (and bone) than the average person. An excellent example of this is the muscularly-developed professional athlete who would be considered overweight but not overfat.

Unfortunately, many individuals are concerned only with how much they weigh rather than how much body fat they have. For your health and fitness, it is not how much you weigh that is important, but how much of your body is lean muscle and bone and how much is fat (adipose tissue). The component of fitness that relates to what percentage of your body weight is fat and what percentage is muscle mass and bone is commonly referred to as body leanness. At West Point, for example, the maximum allowable percent of body fat for men and women cadets is 18 percent and 26 percent respectively. For society in general, the upper range of percent body fat is, regrettably, considerably higher. All individuals would be healthier and would have backs much less likely to suffer the rigors of pain if they maintained a proper level of body leanness. In some instances, individuals develop extremely high levels of body fat. Once men and women reach body fat levels of 30 percent and 35 percent respectively, they are considered to be obese. Obesity is a sure ticket on a train ride to poor health. Such a condition should be avoided without exception.

How To Lose Body Fat

No magic formula exists for fat loss. The only sound method for losing fat is to expend more calories or energy than you consume. As a process, maintaining body leanness can be viewed as the end product of two antagonistic forces on a scale (Table 6-2).

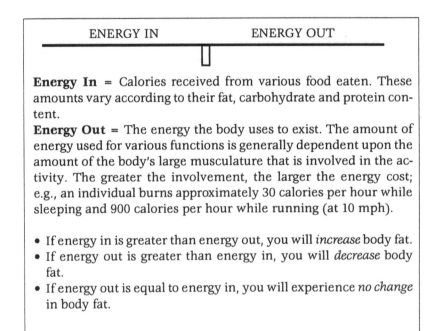

ENERGY IN   ENERGY OUT

Energy In = Calories received from various food eaten. These amounts vary according to their fat, carbohydrate and protein content.

Energy Out = The energy the body uses to exist. The amount of energy used for various functions is generally dependent upon the amount of the body's large musculature that is involved in the activity. The greater the involvement, the larger the energy cost; e.g., an individual burns approximately 30 calories per hour while sleeping and 900 calories per hour while running (at 10 mph).

- If energy in is greater than energy out, you will *increase* body fat.
- If energy out is greater than energy in, you will *decrease* body fat.
- If energy out is equal to energy in, you will experience *no change* in body fat.

Table 6-2   The relationship between energy in and energy out

Since a pound of body fat contains approximately 3,500 calories, if you want to lose two pounds per week, your level of energy consumed (in) must be 7,000 fewer calories than the level of energy you expend (out). This negative balance can be achieved in one of three ways: 1) by burning up an additional 7,000 calories per week (via physical activity), 2) by cutting back 7,000 calories on your total weekly caloric intake (dieting), or 3) a combination of both exercising and dieting. The latter alternative is the most feasible, because it does not involve an unreasonable expenditure of either time or self-discipline on your part. Remember the key to weight control is moderation. Don't starve yourself. You didn't raise your percentage of body fat to an unacceptable level overnight, and you won't lower it overnight. Become familiar with caloric values of the foods that are accessible to you. Calorie charts are sold at the checkpoint counters of most grocery stores. Learn the caloric expenditure totals for the various physical activities in which you might participate. Table 6-3 lists the approximate calorie expenditure by individuals of different body weights in selected physical activities. Calculate your approximate total weekly caloric intake. Next, develop a plan for a proper diet and exercise to achieve a one- to two-pound weight loss per week. Remember, maintaining body leanness is your responsibility. Once you attain an acceptable body fat level, you should continue to exercise and eat wisely in order to preserve what you have achieved. You owe it to your spine to make a commitment to good health.

General Suggestions For Losing Body Fat

The number of books in print dealing with how to lose "weight" is only exceeded by books on religion and cookbooks. Most of the diet books tend to offer the reader a relatively painless approach for losing fat. Claims, counterclaims, gimmicks and the like notwithstanding, all sensible weight (fat) control efforts can be summarized in just five words: *EAT LESS AND EXERCISE MORE.* No magic formula. No quick and easy techniques. Just plain old common sense and the willpower to adhere to basic nutritional guidelines. Although any listing of the possible actions you could take to help maintain your body leanness at an acceptable level would be almost endless, we suggest that you consider the following steps for losing body fat.

1. Exercise regularly and vigorously. Exercises and activities involving much of the body's large musculature and lasting for extended periods of time are recommended. If your back or neck pain presently limits the degree to which you feel like exercising, you should strongly consider engaging in physical activities that minimize the stress imposed on your spine (e.g., swimming).
2. Moderation is the key to weight control. Be aware of how much you eat and take sensible steps to eat moderate amounts of food.
3. Eat a balanced diet. Be sure that you get enough of the essential nutrients for good health. The U.S. Department of Agriculture recommends that everyone have a daily serving from the "Basic Four" to assure a balanced diet: 1) meat, fish, poultry and eggs; 2) milk and milk products; 3) vegetables and fruits; 4) bread and cereals.
4. Decrease your caloric intake. If you cut back 100 calories a day (e.g., a single slice of bread) less than your needs, you will lose 10-12 pounds per year.

5. Learn to eat slowly in order to learn to eat less. Put your fork or spoon down on the table between bites of food. Chew your food thoroughly.

6. Limit the portions of food you eat at meals to one average (reasonable) serving.

7. Omit or restrict free fats such as butter, margarine, mayonnaise, and ice cream.

8. Omit or restrict free sweets such as pastries and candy.

9. Eat regular meals. Your total caloric intake affects your weight, but the number of meals you eat per day does not. Do not eliminate breakfast. Physiologically, breakfast is the most important meal of the day. If you want to reduce your caloric intake by cutting down on the size of your meals, reduce your food intake at lunch or dinner.

10. Avoid "empty calories," especially after the dinner meal. Alcohol is a particularly useless and unneeded source of calories.

11. Weigh yourself daily and keep a written record of your weight. Use the same scale each time and weigh yourself at approximately the same time each day.

12. Eliminate foods needlessly high in calories (e.g., cut the fat off of steak, abstain from putting sugar in your coffee or tea, abstain from using sour cream on your potatoes, limit your intake of alcoholic beverages, abstain from using gravy).

13. Minimize all snacking between meals. If you must eat something between meals, try to eat a sensible snack like raw vegetables or fruit.

14. Avoid diets that concentrate on a single nutrient or that omit certain nutrients altogether. Both types of diets are very dangerous, don't work in the long run and should be avoided at all costs.

15. Do not severely limit your caloric intake. Diets in which you ingest fewer than 1,000 calories per day should only be undertaken with the supervision of a physician. Long-term fasting is particularly detrimental to your health.

EXERCISE

Muscles and ligaments are the common denominator of painful backs and necks. As a result, the single most important therapeutic measure in the vast majority of instances of back pain is proper exercise. Unfortunately, it is somewhat difficult to convince back and neck pain sufferers of that fact and to get them to engage in a regular program of exercise.

ACTIVITY	CALORIES BURNED PER HOUR		
	BODY WEIGHT		
	100 LBS	**150 LBS**	**200 LBS**
ARCHERY	180	240	300
BACK PACKING (40 LB PACK)	305	410	515
BADMINTON	255	340	425
BASEBALL	210	280	350
BASKETBALL (HALF COURT)	225	300	375
BICYCLING (10 MPH)	300	480	600
BOWLING	155	210	260
CANOEING (4 MPH)	275	415	560
DANCE, AEROBIC	355	540	625
DANCE, SOCIAL	210	280	350
FENCING	225	300	375
FITNESS CALISTHENICS	235	310	390
FOOTBALL	225	300	375
GOLF (WALKING)	185	250	315
GYMNASTICS	230	310	390
HANDBALL	450	600	750
HIKING	225	300	375
JOGGING (5 1/2 MPH)	490	650	835
MARTIAL ARTS	230	310	390
MOUNTAIN CLIMBING	450	600	750
RACQUETBALL	450	600	750
ROPE JUMPING (CONTINUOUS)	525	700	875
ROWING	615	820	1025
RUNNING	625	900	1125
SAILING	135	180	225
SKATING, ICE	265	350	440
SKATING, ROLLER	265	350	440
SKIING, CROSS COUNTRY	525	700	875
SKIING, DOWNHILL	450	600	750
SOCCER	405	540	575
SOFTBALL (FAST)	210	280	350
SOFTBALL (SLOW)	220	290	370
STRENGTH TRAINING	350	470	560
SWIMMING (FAST LAPS)	420	630	850
SWIMMING (SLOW LAPS)	240	320	400
TABLE TENNIS	180	240	300
TENNIS	315	420	525
VOLLEYBALL	260	350	485
WALKING	160	210	265
WATERSKIING	360	480	600

To fully comprehend the importance of exercise in treating and preventing back or neck pain, you need to understand that much of the strength of your spine does not come from the bones of your spine. On the contrary, the muscles of your spine and the strapping effect of the spine's ligaments provide the foundation of strength for your spine. Muscles and ligaments are affected in a positive way by exercise. Of particular importance is the fact that proper exercise can increase the strength and efficiency of both your lower back muscles and your neck muscles. Exercise also strengthens and firms your abdominal muscles, thereby reducing the level of stress on the posterior structures of your back caused by a weak or protruding stomach. Finally, some exercises are designed to stretch your lower back and leg muscles. By eliminating the tightness in your muscles, stretching exercises often relieve much of the stress with which your spine must deal. Flexible, relaxed muscles are better able to handle the demands for dynamic movements that are frequently placed upon them.

What Exercises Should You Do?

The literature is replete with suggestions on what exercises you should do to treat and prevent back or neck pain. There are almost as many theories as there are different people willing to espouse an opinion on what you should do. In our opinion, any sensible exercise program for back or neck pain will include both stretching and strengthening exercises. Your strengthening regimen should include exercises for your neck, as well as for both your abdominal region and your lower back. Identifying which exercises to do is largely a matter of personal preference. Whatever exercises you select, however, they should be relatively simple to do and should not place any undue stress on your spine.

We recommend performing the six exercises illustrated in Figures 6-7 through 6-12 to develop the flexor muscles of your lower back. An extraordinarily effective exercise for strengthening the extensor muscles of the lumbar region is illustrated in Figure 6-13. Of the two muscle groups, the extensors appear to play a much more critical role in the treatment and prevention of back pain. Unfortunately, very few safe and effective exercises for developing the extensor muscles of the lower back exist. Since no one has been able to determine how to develop the extensor muscles of the lower back, these muscles have been virtually ignored in most therapeutic exercise programs. The extensor exercise we recommend has been shown to be extremely effective in most instances.

Figures 6-14 through 6-19 illustrate six stretching exercises for the lower back, while Figures 6-20 through 6-25 illustrate six exercises for developing your abdominal muscles. Keep in mind that the number of possible stretching and strengthening exercises from which to choose is quite extensive. The exercises included in this Chapter represent those which we have found to work well for individuals with back or neck pain.

Figures 6-7 through 6-12
Exercises to develop the flexor muscles of the lower back

Figure 6-7   Pelvic Tilt

Tighten your stomach and roll the top of your pelvis backward. You should feel the small of your back flatten. Hold for 15 seconds. Practice holding your back flat while sitting, standing and walking.

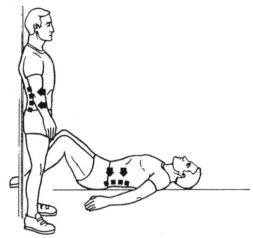

Figure 6-8   Single Knee to Shoulder

Grasp behind your right knee and slowly pull your knee toward your right shoulder. You should feel a gentle stretch on the right side of your back. Hold for 15 seconds. Breathe normally. Alternate with your left knee to your shoulder.

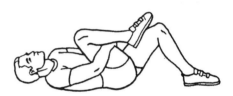

Figure 6-9   Double Knee to Shoulder

Grasp behind both knees; slowly pull them towards your shoulders. You should feel a gentle stretch in the small of your back. Hold for 15 seconds. Breathe normally.

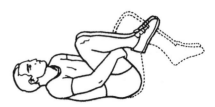

Figure 6-10   Partial Sit-up

Do a pelvic tilt and hold it.
Tuck your chin forward until
your shoulder blades just leave
the floor. You should feel your
stomach muscles working.
Hold for five seconds. Breathe
normally. Slowly lower
yourself back to the floor.

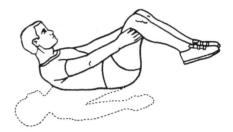

*Figure 6-11   Hip Flexor
Stretch*

Do a pelvic tilt and hold it.
Grasp behind your right knee
and pull it toward your right
shoulder. Flatten your left
thigh against the floor. You
should feel your left buttock
tighten and a stretch at the top
front of your thigh. Hold for 15
seconds. Breathe normally.
Alternate sides.

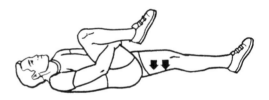

*Figure 6-12   Flexion Resting
Posture*

Lie on your back with your
calves resting on a chair seat.
Completely relax. You should
feel the small of your back
flatten. Remain in this position
for 15 seconds.

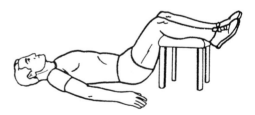

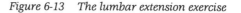

Figure 6-13   The lumbar extension exercise

- This exercise involves two individuals—an exerciser and a training partner.
- Initially, the exerciser assumes a supine position (Figure 16-3a).
- The exercise begins by having the training partner raise both of the exerciser's legs as far as they can go up to a 90 degree maximum (Figure 6-13b).
- The exerciser must keep his/her knees locked throughout the exercise.
- On the command "push" by the training partner, the exerciser extends (pushes) his legs in a downward motion against a force being exerted by the training partner.
- The training partner controls the downward movement of the exerciser's legs, allowing the legs to move in a smooth, steady motion.
- It should take about four seconds for the exerciser to move his/her legs from the starting (90 degree) position to the mid range (45 degree) position (Figure 6-13c).
- Once the exerciser's feet touch the thighs of the training partner, the training partner commands "stop;" the exerciser then stops pushing; and the training partner raises the exerciser's legs back to the starting position.
- The exercise is then repeated; 12-15 repetitions of the exercise should be performed.
- If necessary to keep the exerciser's hips down and the buttocks in constant contact with the floor, the exerciser may need to secure his/her hips to the floor with a strap or belt.

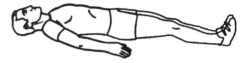

(a)

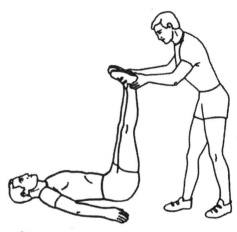

(b)

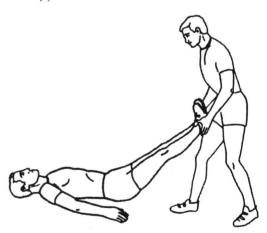

(c)

Figures 6-14 through 6-19
Sample stretching exercises

Figure 6-14

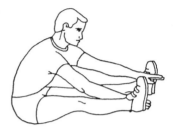

Sit down with your heels 8 to 10 inches apart. With your legs straight, slowly bend forward at your waist. Hold an easy stretch for 10 seconds. Then slightly increase your stretch by bending forward even more. Hold for another 10 seconds.

Figure 6-15

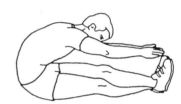

From a standing position, place one leg in front of the other. Keeping both of your legs straight, bend at your waist slowly. Repeat and alternate legs.

Figure 6-16

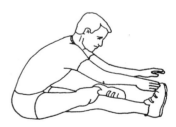

From a sitting position, place one ankle on the knee of your opposite leg. Try to touch your chest to the knee of your straight leg; hold and alternate legs.

Figure 6-17

Sit with your legs stretched out as far as possible without straining. Keep your feet upright and relaxed. Now slowly lean straight forward until you feel a strain on the inside of your legs. Next, stretch your hamstring and back muscles by bending your waist toward your foot. Keep your head up. Hold for 10 seconds; alternate legs.

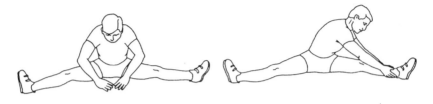

Figure 6-18

Pull the soles of your feet together. With your hands clasped around your feet, slowly pull yourself forward until you feel a stretch in your groin area. Hold an easy stretch for 10 seconds. Slowly increase the stretch as you feel yourself relax. Keep your elbows on the outside of your legs for greater stability.

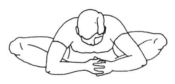

Figure 6-19

Sit on the floor or on a stool with your back straight. Clasp your hands behind your neck. Have a partner stand behind you. Twist your trunk as far as possible while you look over your right shoulder. Have your partner push on your left shoulder and pull gently backward on your right elbow. Hold the position for 10 seconds. Alternate to the other side.

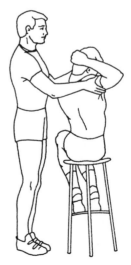

Figure 6-20 through 6-25
Sample exercises to develop the abdominal muscles

Figure 6-20

Stand with your feet shoulder
width apart, your arms
extended up over your head
and your hands clasped
together. Keep your arms close
to your head and slowly bend
to the side, pause, return to the
center, and bend to the other
side. Repeat right, center, left,
center, right, etc. Note: keep
your hips stable.

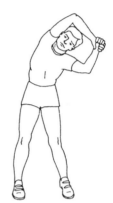

Figure 6-21

On your hands and knees with
your back straight, tuck your
chin to your chest and raise
your back up as you pull in
your stomach muscles (arch
your back like a cat when it
stretches). Relax and repeat.
Note: do not let your back sag
at any time during the exercise.

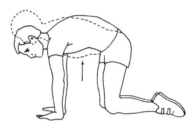

Figure 6-22

From a back-lying position, do
a pelvic tilt. Then straighten
out your left leg and press it flat
to the floor while keeping your
knee rigid. Then without using
your hands and arms for
leverage, raise your
straightened leg as high as you
can until you feel a tightness in
your thigh. After your leg is as
high as you can comfortably
raise it, hold for a count of five.
Then, while you keep your knee
straight, slowly let your leg
return to the floor. Relax, then
repeat with the other leg.
Alternate legs for 10 repetitions.

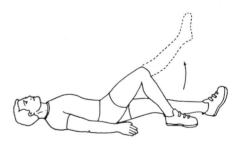

Figure 6-23

Assume a back-lying position with your knees bent and your feet flat on the floor. Your hands may rest on your shoulders or your fingers may be interlocked behind your back. Slowly curl your head toward your knees and continue curling up until your elbows touch your knees.

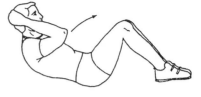

Figure 6-24

Assume a back-lying position with your arms held out at your shoulders. Slowly raise your left leg up (toes pointed) and lower it across your body toward your right hand. If this is too difficult, touch the floor at your waist level or above. Slowly return your leg to a straight-up position and lower it to the floor. Repeat with your right leg, left, right, etc. Note: Keep your back, head and shoulders in contact with the floor as much as possible during the exercise.

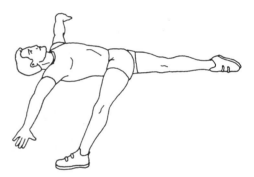

Figure 6-25

Sit with your legs together, toes pointed and hands on your shoulders. Twist your trunk to the right, and continue twisting for four counts while you look over your right shoulder. Repeat to your left, right, left, etc. Note: Do not let your hips turn while you do the exercise. You are in a seated rather than a standing position to stabilize your hips so they cannot assist with the twisting action of your trunk.

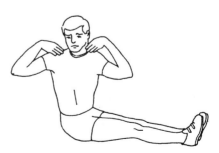

How Should You Organize Your Exercise Program?

Although there are no set ways of organizing an exercise program for treating and preventing back or neck pain, several guidelines exist to help you increase the levels of safety, efficiency and effectiveness of your therapeutic exercise program.

Before beginning your exercise program, you should consult a physician to make sure that the exercises won't aggravate your condition. This caution is particularly important if you are experiencing severe pain.

The schedule of when and how long to do each exercise varies somewhat from individual to individual. Common sense dictates that you should stretch before and after doing the strengthening exercises. If you're performing traditional calisthenic-type stretching and strengthening exercises, you should establish an appropriate order for doing the exercises. The number of repetitions and sets you should perform of each exercise, how many times a day you should exercise and how many times a week you should work out also vary according to your personal perspective of "how much exercise is too much." A point to keep in mind regarding a general philosophy towards exercising is that more (exercise) is not necessarily better.

We recommend performing a single set of 10-12 repetitions of each exercise, three times a week (on alternative days)—unless you're currently suffering from back or neck pain. In that instance, you may need or want to work out every day. Whatever the "quantitative recipe" you finally decide is best for your needs, remember that exercise is not a contest. Don't focus on how much you lift or how many repetitions you can do of a particular exercise. Just perform the program in the proper fashion. If you exercise properly, there are no losers.

BACK PROBLEMS PARTICULAR TO WOMEN

There are some problems relating to back pain that only women have. A noninclusive list of these problems includes menstruation, pregnancy and postnatal back.

Menstruation

In some instances, just before a woman's menstrual period begins, her uterus puts extra pressure on her back because the uterine walls become heavier with the buildup of the lining of the walls. As a result, menstrual periods almost always make a low back condition worse. In addition, most women tend to retain extra fluids throughout their body during the time of their menstrual period. The extra fluids often cause a weight gain of three to ten pounds. More often than not, the extra weight is carried in the stomach. This extra weight produces even more stress on the lower back.

If you experience an increase in low back pain or a substantial weight gain during your menstrual period, we recommend that you eat a high protein diet for approximately ten days, commencing five days before the start of your period. A diet high in protein tends to lessen fluid retention. To minimize the level of stress placed on your lower back by your heavier-than-normal stomach, it is important that you develop very strong abdominal muscles. There is additional nutritional evidence that your diet at this time should also include foodstuffs high in iron and roughage. Nutritionists suggest that such a diet should help give you better control over your abdominal muscles.

One final note on this subject involves the use of tampons. Although the use of tampons causes no trouble for most women, some women cannot use tampons of any kind because they cause back pain. If you're experiencing back pain during your menstrual period, you should consider switching to sanitary napkins. Each individual's level of sensitivity to intrauterine devices (e.g., tampons, diaphragms, IUDs) is different. If you're suffering from low back pain during your menstrual period, you should check out every possibility.

Pregnancy

Pregnancy more often than not causes back pain in expectant mothers as they approach the end of their term. This pain is essentially the result of the mechanical forward adjustment of a pregnant woman's spine which occurs as her increased size shifts her center of gravity forward. As a result, her lower back is forced to deal with greater than normal stresses. In addition, a pregnant woman also must confront the problems caused by mechanical changes in her sacroiliac and other joints. These changes are produced by her body's release of a hormone called relaxin. Relaxin loosens the pelvic ligaments as a precursor to permitting her baby's head to move more easily through her pelvic canal during birth. Like all adjustments to proper body mechanics, these changes place further stress on the pregnant woman's lower back. Coupled with the gradual lessening of her control over her abdominal muscles (the anterior muscles of the back), it is little wonder that back pain is prevalent among expectant mothers.

The program to prevent or at least minimize back pain for expectant mothers is threefold. First, a pregnant woman should strengthen her lower back and abdominal muscles as much as possible. Before commencing her exercise program, an expectant mother should consult her physician to determine an exercise regimen to follow. Second, an expectant mother should be particularly sensitive to proper body mechanics and adhere to them at all times. Finally, an expectant mother should include extra periods of rest (lying down) in her schedule in order to reduce the cumulative amount of stress in her lower back.

Postnatal Back

Right after a woman has given birth, her pelvic ligaments are loosened, the strength of her abdominal muscles is normally quite low and her lower back muscles are usually both tightened and fatigued from the previous months of dealing with the extra stress that was placed upon them. Along with the immediate need to perform the physical demands of carrying, lifting and lowering a new addition to her family, the lowered physical state of a woman in the postnatal period can have catastrophic effects on her back. The solution is similar to the proposed recommendations for dealing with the low back demands of pregnancy. In order to keep the degeneration of her physical state during pregnancy to a minimum, a woman should engage in a sensible exercise program prior to giving birth and for as long a period of time as her physician feels is appropriate for her. Once she gives birth, a woman should recommence her exercise program as soon as possible. Unless there were medical complications during delivery (e.g., cesarean section, hemorrhaging), the time to start an exercise program is now. Finally, in order to be able to minimize the physical demands imposed on her back by handling her baby, a woman needs to be aware of and adhere to proper body mechanics at all times. She should learn how to lift, lower and carry her baby in the manner that is least stressful on her spine.

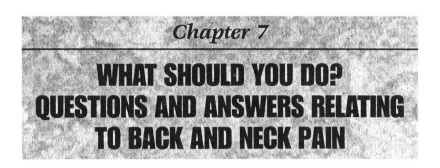

Chapter 7

WHAT SHOULD YOU DO? QUESTIONS AND ANSWERS RELATING TO BACK AND NECK PAIN

"No question is ever settled until it is settled right."
—Ella Wheeler Wilcox

This chapter is devoted to answering some of the questions concerning back and neck pain that we've encountered over the years. Since individuals with back or neck pain tend to have similar problems, chances are that the information presented in this chapter will highlight many points concerning spine pain that have been discussed in detail elsewhere in this book.

Q: *Why do healthy people get back and neck pain?*

A: Unfortunately, it is "normal" for healthy young people to have back or neck pain at some time. In fact, almost everyone has experienced or will experience back or neck pain during their lifetime. About one-half of the working force is unable to go to work because of back or neck pain at some time in their lives. There are several factors that may predispose an otherwise healthy person to back or neck pain. These include the effects of poor posture and excessive weight, pregnancy, overuse injuries and poor flexibility and tight hamstring muscles. Sleeping is another significant factor in back and neck pain that normal healthy people get.

Q: *What are the primary clues for determining the cause of back or neck pain?*

A: The clues are: the location of your pain, the precipitating event that caused your pain, when your back or neck hurts and what makes the pain in your back or neck increase or decrease.

Q: *When should one see a doctor about back or neck pain?*

A: If your back or neck pain shows signs of being more than a minor problem, such as severe, recurrent or chronic pain, you should see a doctor. Also, if you have persistent pain down one of your arms or legs or if there is weakness in one of your arms or legs or bowel or bladder dysfunction, you should contact a doctor.

Q: *What is the process a doctor goes through in evaluating your back or neck pain?*

A: Your doctor should proceed in an organized step-by-step fashion in the evaluation of your back or neck pain. This starts with a good history of your problem, which will answer the questions who, what, where, when, and why. A physical exam is then performed and x-rays and other studies may then be ordered. Regular x-rays are usually the initial test used to evaluate the bones of your spine, just as they are used to evaluate the bones elsewhere in your body. Other x-ray studies such as computerized tomography (CT scan), magnetic resonance imaging (MRI), a bone scan or a myelogram are also sometimes used in the evaluation of back or neck pain. Blood tests are also occasionally ordered in the evaluation of back and neck pain. All of these tests, however, should complement and not replace a good history of your back or neck pain and a thorough physical examination.

Q: *How much of what is known about back pain applies to neck pain?*

A: Quite a bit. Anatomically speaking, your neck is simply an extension of your spine. Some neck problems, however, are different in both quality and kind from back problems.

Q: *What is the best drug for back or neck pain?*

A: Historically, the most widely used drug has been aspirin. Aspirin acts as both a pain killer and as an anti-inflammatory medicine to reduce back or neck pain. The recommended approach for an adult when spinal pain initially strikes is to take two or three aspirin every four hours. Anyone who is sensitive to aspirin, has bleeding tendencies or gastrointestinal problems should be careful taking aspirin and other anti-inflammatory medicines.

There are a number of other anti-inflammatory medicines available without a prescription and a number that are available with a prescription. Tylenol is another commonly used non-prescription mild pain relieving medicine. Tylenol, however, is not an anti-inflammatory medicine and therefore probably will not do as well as aspirin or other anti-inflammatory medicines when a component of the pain problem is inflammation.

Q: *What are natural painkillers?*

A: Our bodies produce their own painkillers, called endorphins. The natural version of morphine, endorphins are chemicals released by the brain to dull pain.

Q: *Is DMSO an effective agent for the treatment of back or neck pain?*

A: DMSO is an acronym for dimethyl sulfoxide, a substance that has been used to treat animals (particularly horses) for many years. We don't recommend it, and its benefits have not been documented. Fortunately, its usage hit its peak in the late seventies and early eighties and appears to be on a dramatic downswing.

Q: *What are the most common injuries to the spine?*

A: The most common injuries of the spine are not injuries to the bone or discs but rather injuries to the ligaments (sprains) and muscles (strains). The mechanism of sprained ligaments and strained muscles in the spine are similar to the mechanisms of injuries that occur elsewhere in the body. For example, athletes can strain a leg muscle running or twist and sprain their ankle ligaments, just as they can strain a back muscle or sprain the ligaments in their backs.

Q: *What is a "ruptured" or "slipped" disc?*

A: Many terms are used to discuss disc injuries including ruptured, slipped, bulging, herniated and degenerative. Each term is actually an accurate description of what has happened to the disc. The discs are flat circular structures between the vertebra and the back and the neck. Discs are made of a cartilage material similar in consistency to rubber and they function as the shock absorbers of the spine. If they are injured or degenerate or "rupture" or "slip", etc., they can be a source of pain in the back and can cause pressure on nerves that are exiting from the spinal cord.

Q: *Who is more likely to suffer from a herniated disc, men or women?*

A: Men. Men, for whatever reason, are also more likely than women to undergo surgery for back conditions of equal severity.

Q: *What is sciatica?*

A: Sciatica is pain caused from irritation or pressure on the sciatic nerve. Sciatica usually starts in your lower back and travels along the course of the sciatic nerve through your buttocks and the back of your leg to your foot. The pain is usually sharp and intense and can be an electric type shooting pain. If the sciatic nerve becomes irritated or pinched enough, numbness or weakness can result. The usual cause of sciatica is an injury or problem with the disc.

Q: *What is spinal stenosis?*

A: Spinal stenosis is a term used to describe narrowing of the spinal canal. Any condition that narrows the spinal canal is, in effect, spinal stenosis. The term spinal stenosis, however, usually refers to the narrowing of the spinal canal that is associated with degenerative arthritis and degenerative discs. Most patients with spinal stenosis are over the age of 50. The diagnosis is made by a history and physical exam, regular x-rays and special studies such as a CT scan or MRI.

Q: *When should an individual return to work after an acute bout of back or neck pain?*

A: Unfortunately, there is no set answer to this question. On one hand, you don't want to delay returning to your normal life-style any longer than is necessary. On the other hand, you don't want to aggravate or prolong your condition needlessly by returning to work too soon. Ultimately, your decision should be based on your doctor's advice and your own assessment of your pain.

Q: *What are the chances that an individual who has suffered back or neck pain previously will have another bout?*

A: The chances are very good. Statistically, the chances are 60-70 percent that you will have a second bout of back pain within two years of your initial bout. If you strengthen and stretch the muscles supporting the spine, your chances of suffering another bout will be greatly reduced.

Q: *Does your mind play a role in treating back or neck pain?*

A: Most definitely. Your mind and your body work together when it comes to pain. By cooperating consciously with your treatment and by believing in your mind's healing powers, you can have a significant effect on your spine. The key is to avoid allowing a negative attitude devastate your life.

Q: *What is the approximate incidence of psychosomatic back or neck pain?*

A: The number of individuals who have back or neck pain of a nonorganic nature has been estimated to be as high as 40-50 percent of all those suffering from back or neck pain. You should keep in mind that the pain suffered by someone with psychosomatic back or neck pain is every bit as "real" as the pain suffered by someone with pain caused by trauma.

Q: *What kind of doctor should someone with back or neck pain see for treatment?*

A: Initially, you should see your family doctor. Your doctor may then refer you to a specialist—an orthopedic surgeon, a neurosurgeon or a rheumatologist. Chiropractors have also been a popular personal choice for many people who suffer from back or neck pain.

Q: *Can chiropractors help back and neck pain?*

A: Chiropractors are licensed health care specialists who utilize spinal manipulation as their primary means of therapy. They also typically use many other non surgical therapies such as heat/cold therapy, massage, and exercise. They generally enjoy wide popularity in the United States and other countries.

Q: *Is acupuncture an effective treatment for back or neck pain?*

A: Acupuncture appears to work for some patients, some of the time. Until research provides a documented answer regarding its benefits and risks, we don't recommend it.

Q: *Should x-rays be taken whenever someone has back or neck pain?*

A: The use of x-rays for individuals with minor back or neck problems should be minimal, if they are used at all. Some physicians use x-rays in these situations merely to assure the patient. No practical information is provided by x-rays in cases of minor back or neck pain. In more serious cases of back or neck pain-related complaints, x-rays serve a useful function.

Q: *What is an MRI?*

A: Magnetic resonance imaging (MRI) is the most recently developed of the various types of studies used in the evaluation of the spine and other parts of the body. The images created by MRI are made using magnetic fields that do not produce radiation exposure. MRI shows not only the bones but the soft tissues of the spine and is especially valuable in helping to evaluate disc problems.

Q: *What is a myelogram?*

A: A myelogram is an x-ray taken after a clear, water-soluble solution (somewhat misnamed as a dye) is injected into the watery, fluid-containing sac surrounding the nerves of the spine. This solution obstructs the passage of x-rays and enables the spinal canal to be outlined in such a way as to reveal anything causing substantial pressure on the nerve roots.

Q: *What does the term "conservative treatment" mean?*

A: Traditionally, this term means nonsurgical treatment. Frankly, we would like to think that all back and neck therapy—surgical and nonsurgical alike—is based on a considered, somewhat cautious perspective. Accordingly, nonsurgical treatment should be rightfully referred to as nonoperative or nonsurgical therapy.

Q: *Is there such a thing as risk-free surgery?*

A: No. Although in most spinal operations there is a small chance that significant problems will develop, there is always some risk involved.

Q: *Would you recommend spinal fusion for back pain diagnosed as idiopathic in nature?*

A: No. All too often, fusion either fails to relieve the symptoms for which it is performed, or it actually makes them worse. In general, we would recommend fusion only to correct documented instability present in the spine, such as may occur as the consequences of trauma or from certain developmental changes or congenital defects.

Q: What is the best sleeping surface for someone with back or neck pain?

A: It is difficult and impossible to say with certainty that any single or specific sleeping surface is the best for everyone. Considering that we spend about eight hours a day or one-third of our total lives sleeping or trying to sleep, it should be apparent to us the importance of a good night's sleep, especially if you have back or neck pain. When viewed from the side, the spine is not straight. Therefore, it is hard to imagine that sleeping on a rigid, flat surface could be comfortable or beneficial for your spine. It certainly makes sense that a mattress and pillow that conform to the shape of your spine and support but distribute uniformly the pressures on your back, neck and different body parts would be ideal.

We have been very impressed with the Tempur-Pedic products and would encourage you to read further about them in Chapter 5.

Q: What is the best position for lying in bed for someone with a sore back?

A: In general, you should lie either on your side with your hips and knees bent or on your back, again with your hips and knees bent. The one position that you should definitely avoid is lying on your stomach.

Q: Should a person with back pain use a waterbed?

A: Some backs like waterbeds, some don't. The only hard-and-fast rule is to use what works for you.

Q: What does heat do for someone with back or neck pain?

A: No one is absolutely certain what heat does. What is certain is that heat helps to soothe your pain. In turn, the continuous cycle of muscle spasm causing pain, causing more muscle spasm, etc. is often broken by the application of heat. It is not known whether or not this change occurs because heat blocks the transmission of pain or because heat causes circulatory changes under the skin.

Q: What kind of heat should someone with back or neck pain use to treat the pain?

A: As long as it isn't too hot and doesn't damage the skin, any form of heat is acceptable. An electric heating pad is as good as anything.

Q: What is traction?

A: As it relates to treating back pain, traction is a form of back therapy in which the upper and lower parts of your body are pulled in opposite directions in order to ease your back pain. In treating neck pain, the neck is "stretched out" by pulling the base of your skull from your upper body. Less weight is used for cervical (neck) traction than lumbar (low back) traction. There are a number of theories as to how traction reduces back or neck pain or pain from pinched nerves. For some people, traction provides relief; for others, it does not and may even aggravate the pain. Home traction units are available. At least initially, traction should only be performed under the supervision of a physical therapist or qualified medical professional.

Q: What is the best sport or exercise for someone who has neck or back pain?

A: Choose an activity that you enjoy doing and one in which the pleasure you derive from your participation exceeds any pain that may result. Obviously, you shouldn't engage in any sport that places undue stress on your neck or back. For example, soccer and touch football shouldn't be on your weekend activity schedule if you have severe neck or back pain.

Q: What is a pelvic tilt exercise?

A: Essentially, the pelvic tilt is an exercise that involves a movement very similar to the pelvic motion basic to lovemaking. This exercise is designed to strengthen your anterior spine structure and to stretch the posterior spine structure.

Q: Can vibrating chairs, beds or hand massagers help relieve back or neck pain?

A: Massaging agents (chairs, beds or hand-held vibrator) can certainly soothe your back or neck and relax tense muscles. Massage tends to have the same effect as the application of heat.

Q: Can an individual with chronic back pain ever be able to have a satisfying sex life?

A: As you well know, a satisfactory sex life is no small achievement, even for someone with a pain-free back. If you have back pain, you are going to have to be aware of certain adjustments that you may have to make in your lovemaking techniques if you are to have a satisfying love life. Refer to Chapter 6 for a discussion of some of the factors that should be considered.

Q: *It is possible that an automobile accident can produce an injury to someone's back or neck that won't manifest itself until months or years later?*

A: This almost never happens. If your pain doesn't appear within 48 hours or so after the accident, chances are that the accident is not the cause of your back or neck pain.

Q: *Does a difference in the lengths of a person's legs cause back pain?*

A: Difference in leg lengths up to three-eighths of an inch is normal and differences as much as three-fourths of an inch usually have no effect on your back.

Q: *Can the Tempur-Pedic Swedish Mattress and Neck Pillow really help someone with back or neck pain?*

A: Depending upon the nature and severity of the back or neck problem, the Tempur-Pedic Swedish pressure-relieving Mattress and Neck Pillow can be as effective or more effective than pain-relieving drugs. Used in conjunction with the common sense attitude toward back and neck pain outlined in this book, the Tempur-Pedic Swedish Mattress and Neck Pillow can be an integral part of the therapeutic program.

Q: *If I have an antique or odd-sized bed, can I get a custom-sized Tempur-Pedic Swedish Mattress to fit my bed?*

A: Yes. Tempur-Pedic, Inc. frequently gets requests for custom-sized Tempur-Pedic Swedish Mattresses and they are more than happy to accommodate your request.

For more information you can call 1-800-886-6466 or write:

Tempur-Pedic, Inc.,
848G Nandino Blvd.
Lexington, KY 40511

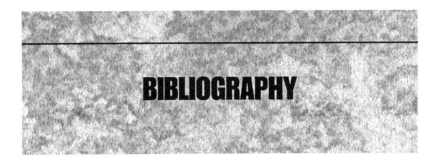

BIBLIOGRAPHY

Anderson, B.J. "A Quantitative Study of Back Loads in Lifting." *Spine 1* (1976): 1978-85.

Basmajian, J.V. *Grant's Method of Anatomy.* 8th ed. Baltimore: Williams and Wilkins Company, 1975.

Becker, F.R., James Wilson and J.A. Gehweiler. *The Anatomical Basis of Medical Practice.* Baltimore: Williams and Wilkins Company, 1971.

Benson, Herbert. *The Relaxation Response.* New York: William Morrow and Company, 1975.

Burkholtz, Herbert. "Pain: Solving the Mystery." *The New York Times Magazine* 27 September 1987: 16-19, 32-35.

Cailliet, Rene. *Low Back Pain Syndrome.* 2nd ed. Philadelphia: F.A. Davis Company, 1974.

Caldwell, A.B. and C. Chase. "Diagnosis and Treatment of Personality Factors in Chronic Low Back Pain." *Clinical Orthopedics* 129 (1977): 141-49.

Chaffin, D.B. "Human Strength Capacity and Low Back Pain." *Journal of Occupational Medicine* 16 (1974): 248.

Cousins, Norman. *Anatomy of an Illness as Perceived by the Patient.* New York: Bantam Books, 1981.

Finneson, Bernard E. *Low Back Pain.* Philadelphia: J.B. Lippincott Company, 1981.

Fordyce, W.E., et al. "Pain Management and Pain Behavior." *Pain* 18 (1984): 53-69.

Friedmann, Lawrence W. and Lawrence Galton. *Freedom From Backaches.* New York: Pocket Books, 1984.

Hoeger, Warner W. *Lifetime Physical Fitness and Wellness.* Englewood, CO: Morton Publishing Company, 1986.

Hoppenfeld, Stanley. *Physical Examination of the Spine and Extremities.* New York: Appleton-Century-Crofts, 1976.

Isselbacher, K.J., R.D. Adams, E. Braunwald, R.G. Petersdort and J.D. Wilson, eds. *Principles of Internal Medicine.* New York: McGraw-Hill Book Company, 1980.

Jayson, M.I.V. *The Lumbar Spine and Back Pain.* Tunbridge Wells, England: Pitman Medical Publisher, 1980.

Krusen, Frank H., ed. *Handbook of Physical Medicine and Rehabilitation.* 2nd. ed. Philadelphia: W.B. Sauder Company, 1971.

Lettvin, Maggie. *Maggie's Back Book.* Boston: Houghton Mifflin Company, 1976.

Licht, Sidney, ed. *Rehabilitation and Medicine.* Baltimore: Waverly Press, 1968.

Lonetto, Richard and Gayle Kumchy. *Back to Normal.* Toronto: Doubleday and Company, 1986.

Macnab, Ian. *Backache.* Baltimore: Williams and Wilkins Company, 1977.

Masters, W.H. and V. Johnson. *Human Sexual Inadequacy.* Boston: Little, Brown and Company, 1970.

Melzack, R. and P.D. Wall. "Pain Mechanisms: A New Theory." *Science* 150 (1965): 971-79.

Mountcastle, Vernon B. *Medical Physiology.* 14th ed. St. Louis, MO: C.V. Mosby Company, 1980.

Nechemson, A.L. "The Lumbar Spine—An Orthopaedic Challenge." *Spine* 1 (1976): 59.

Norton, P.L. and T. Brown. "The Immobilizing Efficiency of Back Braces." *Journal of Bone Joint Surgery* 39A (1957): 104-13.

Osborne, D. and T. Maruta. "Sexual Adjustment and Chronic Back Pain." *Medical Aspects of Human Sexuality* 14 (1980): 104-13.

Pelletier, Kenneth R. *Mind as Healer, Mind as Slayer.* New York: DEU, 1977.

Peterson, James A. and Susan L. Peterson. *The Sexy Stomach.* West Point, NY: Leisure Press, 1983.

Root, Leon and Thomas Kiernan. *Oh, My Aching Back.* New York: New American Library, 1985.

Sarno, John. *Mind Over Back Pain.* New York: Berkley Books, 1986.

Strauss, Richard H. ed. *Sports Medicine and Physiology.* Philadelphia: W.B. Saunders Company, 1979.

Tarlov, Edward and David D'Costa. *Back Attack.* Boston: Little, Brown and Company, 1985.

Toufexis, A. "The Aching Back." *Time* 14 July 1980: 30-38.

White, Augustus A. *Your Aching Back.* New York: Bantam Books, 1983.

White, A.A. and M.M. Panjabi. "The Clinical Biomechanics of Spine Pain" (Chapter 6). *The Clinical Biomechanics of the Spine.* Philadelphia: J.B. Lippincott, 1978.

Williams, Paul C. *Low Back and Neck Pain.* Springfield, IL: Charles C. Thomas, Publisher, 1974.

_____. *The Lumbosacral Spine—Emphasizing Conservative Management.* New York: McGraw-Hill Book Company, 1965.

INDEX

(page numbers in italics denote illustrations)

ABOUT THE AUTHORS

James H. Wheeler, M.D., FAAOS, FACS, is an orthopedic surgeon specializing in sports medicine and athletic injuries who is presently in private practice in Marion, North Carolina. A graduate of Marquette University in Milwaukee, Wisconsin, Jim attended the Medical College of Wisconsin and did his orthopedic surgery residency training in Grand Rapids, Michigan. Following residency, Jim served eight years in the United States Army, in Germany (1981-1985) at the Landstuhl Army Regional Medical Center and at the United States Military Academy at West Point (1985-1989). He is board certified by the American Board of Orthopedic Surgery, a fellow of the American Academy of Orthopedic Surgeons and a fellow of the American College of Surgeons. He is also a member of the American Orthopedic Society for Sports Medicine, the Arthroscopy Association of North America and the American College of Sports Medicine.

James A. Peterson, Ph.D., FACSM, is a sports medicine specialist who resides in Monterey, California. The author of 43 books and over 100 published articles, Jim previously served as the Director of Sports Medicine for StairMaster Sports/Medical Products, Inc. (1990-1995) and as a professor on the Department of Physical Education faculty at the United States Military Academy at West Point (1970-1990). A graduate of the University of California at Berkeley, Jim is a Fellow of the American College of Sports Medicine.

It was at West Point, New York that the authors met, worked together professionally, became friends and furthered their interest in the treatment and prevention of sports injuries. Their common interest in the treatment and prevention of back pain in the West Point cadets and staff let to the first edition of this book. Their continued interest in the treatment of back and neck pain has led to this second edition and is discussed further in the Introduction.